Rebeh Bougossa
Fatma Larbi
Chawki Loussaief

Carbapenem-resistant Enterobacteriaceae urinary tract infections

Rebeh Bougossa
Fatma Larbi
Chawki Loussaief

Carbapenem-resistant Enterobacteriaceae urinary tract infections

ScienciaScripts

Imprint

Any brand names and product names mentioned in this book are subject to trademark, brand or patent protection and are trademarks or registered trademarks of their respective holders. The use of brand names, product names, common names, trade names, product descriptions etc. even without a particular marking in this work is in no way to be construed to mean that such names may be regarded as unrestricted in respect of trademark and brand protection legislation and could thus be used by anyone.

Cover image: www.ingimage.com

This book is a translation from the original published under ISBN 978-620-6-70858-2.

Publisher:
Sciencia Scripts
is a trademark of
Dodo Books Indian Ocean Ltd. and OmniScriptum S.R.L publishing group

120 High Road, East Finchley, London, N2 9ED, United Kingdom
Str. Armeneasca 28/1, office 1, Chisinau MD-2012, Republic of Moldova, Europe
Printed at: see last page
ISBN: 978-620-7-99344-4

Contents

1 INTRODUCTION

urinary tract infection (UTI) is an attack on the urinary tract by one or more micro-organisms, generating an inflammatory response and symptoms of varying nature and intensity depending on the terrain. The importance of this condition lies in its frequency. The increasing frequency worldwide of bacterial resistance to antibiotics complicates the therapeutic management of this pathology, and justifies periodic regional monitoring of the efficacy of these drugs.

The global spread of Enterobacteriaceae producing extended-spectrum β-lactamases has led to an increase in the prescription of carbapenems. The use of carbapenems is accompanied by the emergence of carbapenem-resistant enterobacteria. These strains are very often multi-resistant to most of the antibiotics most frequently used in human medicine, particularly aminoglycosides and fluoroquinolones, which can lead to real therapeutic impasses. This spread is all the more critical because it occurs at a time when the development of new molecules active against Gram-negative bacilli is still limited. As a result, urinary tract infections caused by carbapenem-resistant uropathogens are currently a major public health problem, both worldwide and in France.

We are proposing this study, which aims to :

determine the epidemiological, clinical, biological, therapeutic and evolutionary characteristics of carbapenem-resistant enterobacterial urinary tract infections in our region and

- investigate the factors involved in the selection of these resistant strains.

I. Urinary tract infection

UTI is an attack on all or part of the urinary tract by one or more micro-organisms, which are responsible for an inflammatory reaction. The clinical manifestations of UTIs vary and depend essentially on the patient's condition. Diagnosis is based on the presence of suggestive clinical signs (urinary signs and/or back pain and/or fever) and significant bacteriuria associated with leucocyturia.

1. Types of UTI: cystitis, acute pyelonephritis, male urinary tract infection

1.1. Acute cystitis

It results from an inflammatory response to the adhesion of pathogens to the bladder urothelium. It is manifested by one or more of the following urinary functional signs:

- Burning while urinating
- Pollakiuria (increased frequency of micturition) and urinary urgency
- Other less frequent signs include hypogastric pain, terminal haematuria and cloudy urine.

These urinary signs are isolated. Fever and back pain are absent.

1.2. Acute pyelonephritis

The typical clinical picture combines signs of cystitis which are often inaugural and discreet, or may be absent, with signs of renal parenchymal involvement:

- fever and chills
- pain in the lumbar fossa, often unilateral, radiating downwards towards the external genitalia, spontaneous or provoked by palpation, percussion or shaking of the lumbar fossa.
- digestive signs (vomiting, diarrhoea, abdominal bloating), which are uncommon but sometimes prominent

There are frustrated forms with a simple fever and/or only provoked low back pain, hence the importance of systematically looking for these symptoms in a patient presenting with a picture suggestive of cystitis.

1.3. Male urinary tract infections

Male UTIs are clinically heterogeneous, ranging from mildly symptomatic forms with no fever (known as "cystitis-like") to forms with obvious parenchymal involvement, which may even lead to septic shock. In some forms, prostatic involvement is clinically evident: pelvic pain apart from micturition, tense prostate enlarged and painful on rectal examination, these symptoms can be described as prostatitis.

In other cases, the dominant signs are those of ANP, both clinically and on imaging.

2. Forms according to the presence of risk factors for complications or the presence of complications

The new recommendations for the management of bacterial urinary tract infections in adults from the Société de Pathologie Infectieuse de Langue Française (SPILF) classify UTIs as : uncomplicated UTI, UTI at risk of complication and severe UTI [1].

2.1. Simple UI

These cases exclusively concern young women with no complication risk factors. They include simple cystitis and simple PNA.

2.2. UTI at risk of complication

These are UTIs occurring in patients with at least one risk factor that can make the infection more serious and treatment more complex, and include: cystitis at risk of complication, ANP at risk of complication and UTIs.

- The risk factors for complications of UTIs are :

- any organic or functional abnormality of the urinary tract (bladder residue, reflux, lithiasis, tumour, recent surgery, etc.)

- male sex, due to the frequency of underlying anatomical or functional anomalies

-young child

-pregnancy

- elderly subject :

* patient over 65 with ≥3 criteria of frailty from the Fried classification: (involuntary weight loss in the last year, slow walking speed, low endurance, weakness/fatigue, reduced physical activity).

*or patient over 75

-severe immunodepression

- severe chronic renal insufficiency (clearance <30 ml/min),

Diabetes, even insulin-requiring diabetes, is no longer a risk factor for complications.

2.3. severe UTI

In the case of parenchymal infection, it is important to determine whether the criteria for severity are met:

- sepsis
- septic shock
- an indication for surgical or interventional drainage (excluding simple bladder catheterisation, because of the risk of worsening sepsis perioperatively).

In the case of ANP or MUI, the presence of one of these 3 severity criteria defines a serious form.

II. Carbapenems

1. Definition

Carbapenems are natural or semi-synthetic antibiotics belonging to the beta-lactam family and obtained from *Streptomyces cattleya.*

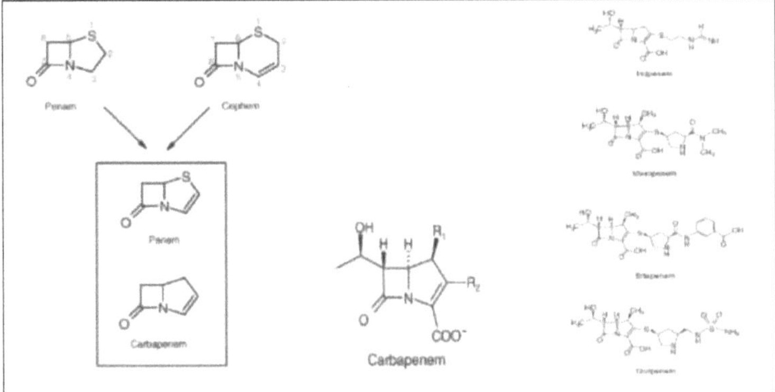

Figure 1: Structure of carbapenems [2].

Four molecules represent this subclass of b-lactam: imipenem, meropenem, ertapenem and doripenem.

In Tunisia, only imipenem and ertapenem are marketed.

2. Mechanism and spectrum of action of carbapenems

Like other ß-lactams, carbapenems exert their bactericidal activity by binding to penicillin binding proteins (PLPs). Unlike cephalosporins and aminopenicillins, which bind mainly to PLP3, carbapenems target PLP1a, 1b and 2, resulting in lysis without prior filamentation and less endotoxin release from Gram-negative bacilli [2] (fig.2).

In enterobacteria, the main porins involved in the passage of antibiotics are those of the OmpF and OmpC families. Any change in the number or activity of these porins can have an immediate impact on resistance to carbapenems [3].

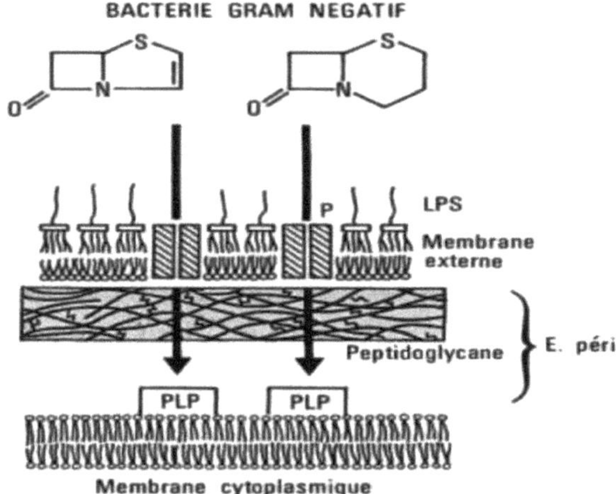

Figure 2: Schematic representation of the wall of gram-negative bacilli [4] PE: Periplasmic space, LPS: Lipopolysaccharides, P: Porins, PLP: Penicillin-binding proteins.

The antibacterial spectrum of carbapenems is broad and virtually the same for all molecules, with the exception of a few differences [2] (Tables I and II).

In fact, all carbapenems are active against gram-positive bacteria, except meticillin-resistant staphylococci and enterococci, but only imipenem retains some activity against *Enterococcus faecalis*. This subclass of antibiotics is active against Enterobacteriaceae, including ESBL-producing strains and high-level cephalosporinase-producing group III strains, as well as *Pseudomonas aeruginosa* and *Acinetobacter baumannii*, with the exception of ertapenem. This is the only carbapenem that cannot be active on *P. aeruginosa* and *Acinetobacter baumannii*. In addition, carbapenems are not active on *Stenotrophomonas maltophilia* (due to the natural production of a metallo-beta-lactamase).

The 4 molecules are highly active on all gram-positive and gram-negative anaerobic bacteria. Their combination with Eamikacin is active against *Nocardia spp.*

Table I: In vitro activity of carbapenems on Gram-negative bacteria [2].

Bacteria	Imipéneme	Meropenem	Doripeneme	Ertapenem
E. coli	0,12/0,25	0,016/0,03	0,03/0,06	< 0,015/s 0,015
E. coli ESBL	0,25/0,5	0,03/0,06	0,03/0,06	0,03/0,25
K. pneumoniae	< 0,06/1	0,03/0,12	0,06/0,12	<0,015/0,12
K. pneumoniae ESBL	0,25/1	0,03/0,12	0,06/0,12	0,06/0,25
Proteus mirabilis	0,5/2	0,06/0,06	0,12/0,25	<0.06/<0,06
Morsanella morsami	2/8	0,12/0,25	0,25/0,5	<0,015/0,03
E. cloacae	0,5/2	0,03/0,06	0,03/0,06	<0,015/0,06
Citrobacter freundii	1/1	0,03/0,06	0,03/0,03	<0,015/0,06
Serratia marcescens	1/2	0,06/0,12	0,12/0,25	0,03/0,12
H. influenzae	0,5/1	0,12/1	0,12/1	0,06/0,25

Moraxella Catarrhalis	0,06/0,12	≤ 0,015/< 0,015	0,12/0,25	0,06/0,25
Salmonella sp	<O,5/<O,5	0,03/0,03	0,06/0,06	< 0,06/<0,06
P. aerusinosa	1/32	0,5/32	0,5/8	> 8/> 8
Acinetobacter baumannii	0,25/0,25	0,25/1	0,25/1	4/> 8
Stenotrophomas maltophilia	> 8/> 8	> 16/> 16	>16/>16	> 8/> 8
Bacteroides frasilis	0,25/1	0,12/1	0,25/1	0,25/1
Prevotella spp	0,03/0,5	0,12/0,25	0,12/0,25	0,25-1
Fusobacterium spp	0,12/1	0,12/0,25	0,12/0,25	0,25/4

Data are MIC50 and MIC90 expressed in mg/l

Table II: In vitro activity of carbapenems on gram-positive bacteria [2].

Bacteria	Imipeneme	Meropenem	Doripenem	Ertapenem
Staphylococcus aureus (MS)	0,06/0,06	0,12/0,12	0,06/0,06	0,12/0,25
S.aureus (MR)	R	R	R	R
Streptoeocus pyogenes	s 0.008/s 0.008	s 0.008/s 0.008	s 0.008/s 0.008	s 0.008/s 0.008
S. agalactiae	0,016/0,016	0,03/0,06	0,016/0,016	0,03/0,06
S. pneumoniae (PeniS)	s 0.06/s0.06	≤0,015/s 0,015	s 0.015/s 0.015	s 0.015/s 0.015
S. pneumoniae(PéniR)	0,5/1	0,5/1	0,5/1	1/2
Enterococcus faecalis	1/4	4/8	4/8	8/32
E. faecium	>8/>8	> 16/> 16	> 16/> 16	> 16/> 16
Listeria monocytogenes	0,03/0,12	0,12/0,12	No data	0,25/0,5
Peptostreptococcus spp.	0,03/0,06	0,12/0,25	0,12/0,25	0,25/4

Data are MIC50 and MIC90 expressed in mg/l

3. Mechanisms of bacterial resistance to carbapenems

The emergence of resistance to carbapenems in bacteria can lead to therapeutic impasses.

The two main mechanisms of carbapenem resistance in Enterobacteriaceae are..:

- The acquisition of genes coding for enzymes capable of hydrolysing carbapenems: carbapenemases

- a qualitative and/or quantitative reduction in bacterial membrane permeability associated with the overexpression of enzymes with very low hydrolytic activity towards carbapenems (production of a cephalosporinase or ESBL coupled with a deficiency or alteration of porins) [3].

3.1. Carbapenemases

3.1.1. Definition

These are beta-lactamases (bacterial enzymes capable of hydrolysing the β-lactam cycle, rendering the antibiotic inactive before it reaches the PLPs) with high hydrolytic activity towards carbapenems [5].

They represent the most important mechanism of resistance from a clinical point of view, as they compromise the efficacy of almost all beta-lactam antibiotics.

3.1.2. Classification

The classification of β-lactamases can be defined according to two properties: functional and molecular. There are several classes of carbapenemases. Each class is designated by a three-letter acronym, such as KPC = *Klebsiella pneumoniae* carbapenemases; NDM = New Delhi metallo-P-lactamases.

• Functional classification [6]

It has undergone numerous modifications since Karen Bush's initial classification in 1988. It currently divides the best-known β-lactamases into four main functional groups (groups 1 to 4), with several sub-groups of group 2 which are differentiated according to the specific substrate group or a profile inhibitor. In this functional classification, carbapenemases are mainly found in functional groups 2f, 3 and 2d (see table III).

Table III: Functional classification of carbapenemases [6].

GROUPES FONCTIONNELS	TYPE D'ENZYME
2f	NMC
	IMI
	SME
	KPC
	GES
3	IMP
	VIM
	GIM
	SPM
	NDM
2d	OXA

• Molecular classification [7]

Ambler and others have classified beta-lactamases on the basis of amino acid sequences into four groups (A to D):

• Class A: serine protease penicillinases, inhibited by clavulanic acid and tazobactam.

• Class B: metallo-enzymes whose active site contains a zinc ion, resistant to clavulanic acid but inhibited by EDTA.

• Class C: cephalosporinases insensitive to clavulanic acid, but inhibited by cloxacillin,

• Class D: oxacillinases that hydrolyse cloxacillin and are only slightly inhibited by clavulanic acid.

In this molecular classification system, carbapenemases are divided into classes A, B and D (Figure 3).

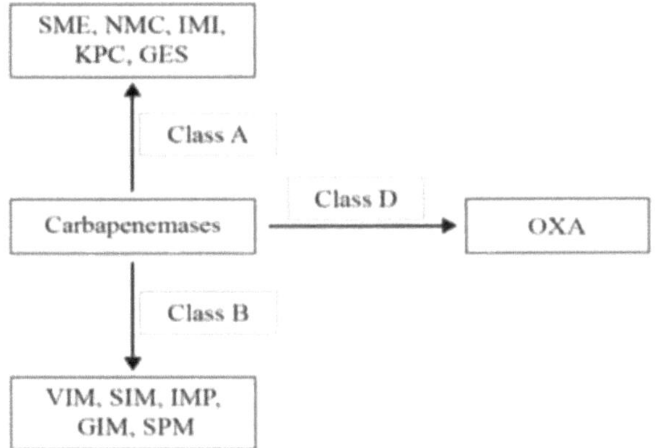

Figure 3: Ambler classification of carbapenemases [7].

3.1.3. Global emergence of carbapenemases

EPCs have rapidly emerged in different parts of the world, making them a truly global epidemic.

Here we present the epidemic outbreaks of the world's main carbapenemases.

❖ *Klebsiella pneumoniae carbapenemase (KPC)*

As its name suggests, KPC is strongly associated with *K. pneumoniae*, but has been found in various enterobacteria such as *Salmonella enterica*, *E. coli* and *K. oxytoca*, as well as in *Pseudomonas aeruginosa* [8].

To date, 19 variants have been identified, but the first identified in the USA in 1996, KPC-2, remains the most common [9]. The countries most affected are the USA, Israel, Greece and Italy [3]. Figure 3 is a map showing the geographical distribution of KPC-producing Enterobacteriaceae worldwide in 2012.

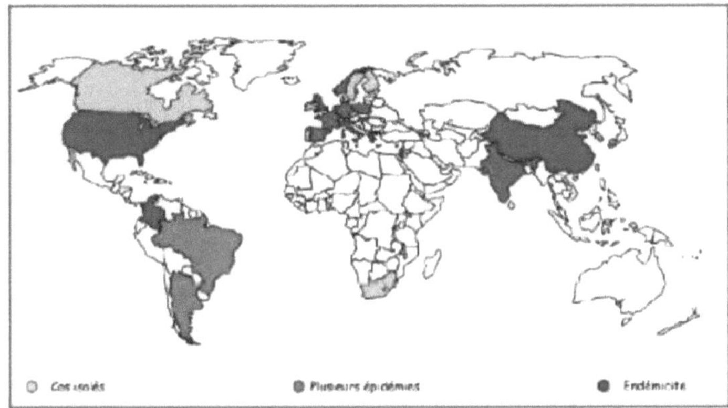

Figure 4: Geographical distribution of KPC-producing Enterobacteriaceae in 2012 [3].

❖ *New Delhi metallo-beta-lactamases (NDM)*

The NDM with the greatest clinical impact is NDM-1, first identified in 2009 in

Sweden in a patient returning from India [10]. Subsequently, this carbapenemase emerged very rapidly around the world. However, this enzyme is more common in the Indian subcontinent (India, Pakistan and Bangladesh) [3] (Figure 5). The rate of faecal colonisation by NDM-1-producing Enterobacteriaceae was 18.5% in a military hospital in Rawalpindi, Pakistan [11]. Widespread environmental dissemination (in water) of various species of NDM-1-producing Enterobacteriaceae has been reported in New Delhi [12].

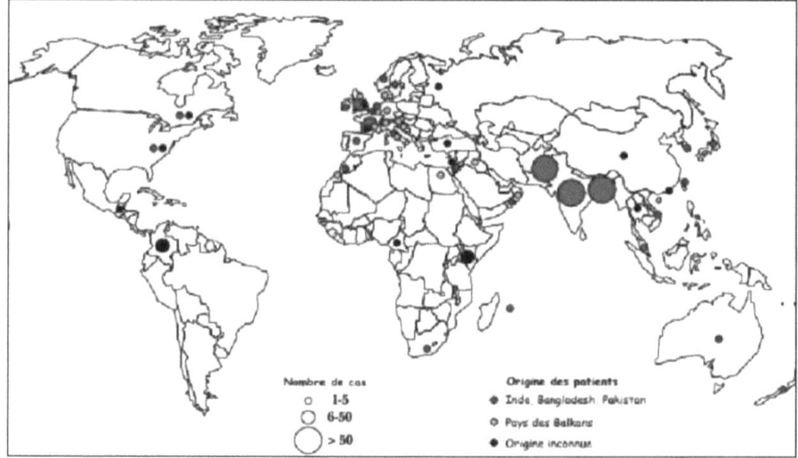

Figure 5: Geographical distribution of NDM-producing Enterobacteriaceae in 2012 [3].

❖ ♦♦ *Oxacillinase-48 (Oxa-48)*

OXA-48 was first isolated in 2003 from a Turkish patient [13], and subsequently spread throughout Turkey, the Middle East and North Africa [3] (Figure 6).

In general, Ambler's class D beta-lactamases or "OXA" (oxacillinases) form a family made up of 256 variants, a small number of which have carbapenemase activity. OXA-48 is not a potent carbapenemase: in the absence of other resistance mechanisms such as other β-lactamases (ESBL or AmpC type), loss of porins or efflux pumps, it causes a slight reduction in sensitivity to carbapenems (low-level resistance), which can make it difficult to detect in the laboratory [14].

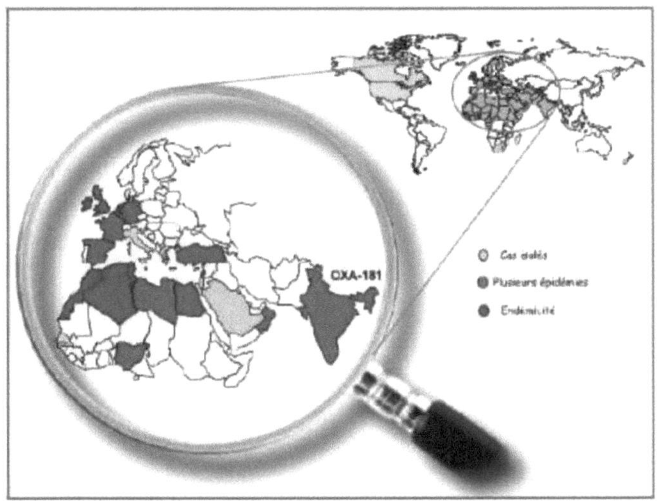

Figure 6: Geographical distribution of OXA-48-producing Enterobacteriaceae in 2012
[3]

3.2. Alteration of penicillin binding proteins (PLPs)

In enterobacteria, certain strains of *Proteus mirabilis* may be resistant to imipenem as a result of alterations to PLPs (through a loss of affinity for PLP2 and a reduction in the quantity of PLP1a). However, this type of mechanism remains very rare [15].

3.3. Association of mechanisms

In enterobacteria, resistance to carbapenems is mainly due to a combination of resistance mechanisms, combining a quantitative or qualitative reduction in the expression of transmembrane proteins known as porins with the production of an enzyme that does not have significant hydrolytic activity towards carbapenems, such as chromosomal or plasmid cephalosporinases, or ESBLs [3].

Initially, this mechanism was described in enterobacterial species that naturally produce a cephalosporinase (*Enterobacter spp, Serratia.spp, Citrobacter freundii, Morganella morganii*, etc.) [16] [17]. More recently, resistance to carbapenems has been observed by combining a cephalosporinase or ESBL with a reduction in porin expression in enterobacterial species that do not naturally express a cephalosporinase (*Klebsiella pneumoniae, Proteus mirabilis, Escherichia coli, Salmonella spp*) [18] [19] [20].

These strains, which are resistant to carbapenems but do not produce carbapenemases, are much less resistant to other families of antibiotics than EPCs.

A combination of mechanisms has been reported for OXA-48 strains [21] , MBLs [22] and more rarely for KPCs [23], which alone already present high levels of resistance to carbapenems.

We conducted a retrospective study during the study period from January 1, 2014 to April 30, 2018. All patients admitted to the wards of the Taher Sfar University Hospital in Mahdia with a diagnosis of carbapenem-resistant Enterobacteriaceae urinary tract infection were included in the study.

I. Data collection

To identify patients with ERC urinary tract infections, we consulted the records of cytobacteriological examinations of urine carried out at the microbiology laboratory of the Taher Sfar University Hospital in Mahdia during the study period.

The epidemiological, clinical, paraclinical, therapeutic and evolutionary characteristics of the patients were collected on a pre-established form (Appendix 1) from the patients' medical records.

II. Inclusion/exclusion criteria

All patients presenting with clinical signs of a urinary tract infection with a cytobacteriological examination of the urine isolating carbapenem-resistant bacteria were included in the study.

Patients with carbapenem-resistant urinary tract colonisation were excluded from the study.

III. Microbiological study

Bacteriological examination and antibiotic susceptibility testing were carried out at the microbiology laboratory of the Taher Sfar University Hospital in Mahdia.

Germ identification was carried out using conventional laboratory techniques.

Antibiotic susceptibility was assessed using the Mueller-Hinton agar diffusion method, in accordance with the recommendations of the Antibiogram Committee of the French Microbiology Society.

IV. Study of risk factors

The following factors were studied as risk factors for the acquisition of ERC urinary tract infections (some of them are included in the literature and the others seem to be associated with a high risk of developing these infections);

S Age

J Gender

J Medical history

J Previous hospitalisation

J History of carriage of carbapenem-resistant bacteria

J Previous use of antibiotics

J Invasive procedures (urinary catheterisation, etc.)

J Notion of proximity to a patient colonised by BRC...

V. Statistical analysis

The data were entered and analysed using SPSS version 24 software.

Qualitative variables were expressed as percentages and headcounts.

Quantitative variables were expressed as mean and standard deviation.

For the analytical study, we used the chi^2 (X^2) or Fischer test to compare percentages and Student's t-test to compare means.

A value of $p < 0.05$ was considered significant.

I. Epidemiological data

1. Prevalence

During the period of our study, 7362 patients hospitalised at the Taher Sfar Mahdia University Hospital had at least one positive urine cytobacteriological examination isolating enterobacteria. In 34 cases (0.46%), the bacteria were resistant to carbapenems. Bacteriuria were asymptomatic in 11 cases (32.4%) and urinary tract infection in 23 cases (67.6%).

2. Annual breakdown

The average annual incidence of carbapenem-resistant uropathogenic urinary tract infections in the various departments was 5.75 cases/year, with extremes ranging from 2 to 10 cases/year (Figure 7). The highest number of cases was recorded in 2015.

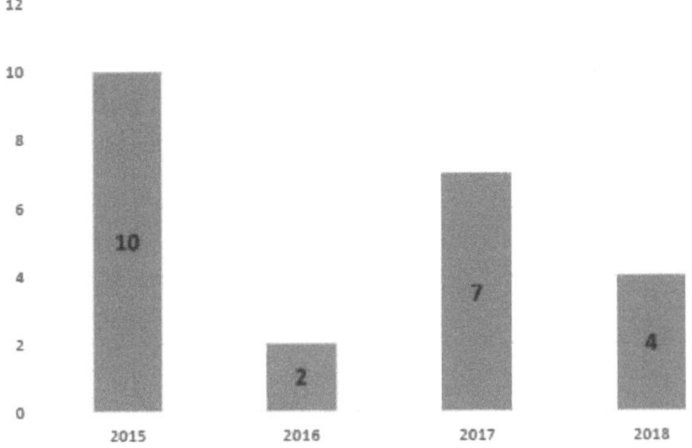

Figure 7: Annual distribution of carbapenem-resistant uropathogenic UTIs

3. Breakdown by department

During the period of our study, carbapenem-resistant Enterobacteriaceae UTIs were identified in six departments (Figure 8). Polyvalent intensive care and urology departments topped the list. In fact, 47.8% and 26.1% of cases were recorded in the latter two departments respectively.

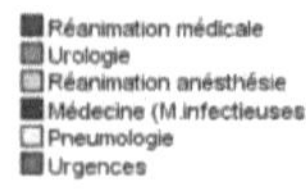

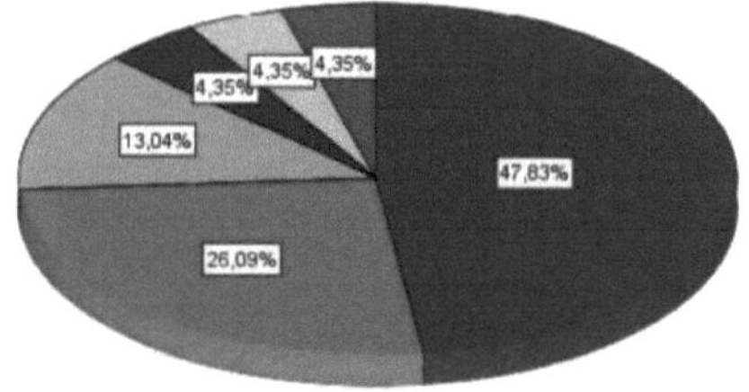

Figure 8: Breakdown of patients by department

4. Age and sex

Our patients were divided into 10 men (43.5%) and 13 women (56.5%) with a sex ratio (M/F) of 0.77.

The mean age of the patients was 57.35 +/- 17.01 years, with extremes ranging from 18 to 80 years. Ten patients (43.5%) were aged between 56 and 65 and eight (34.8%) were aged over 65 (Figure 9).

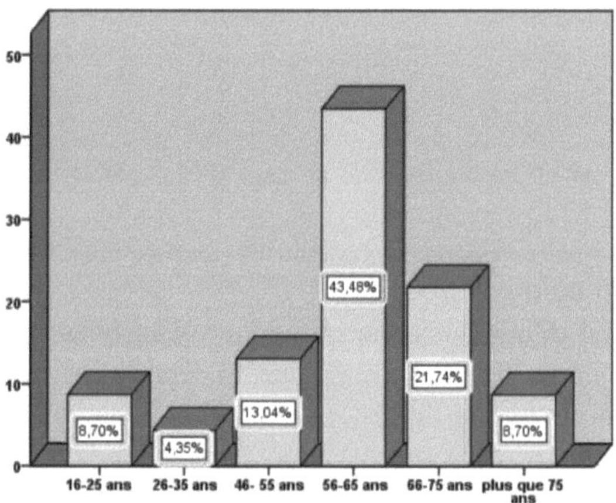

Figure 9: Breakdown of patients by age group

Men were older than women (62.8±13.6 versus 53.2±18.6 years).

5. Comorbidities

One or more pathological histories were present in 21 patients.

Comorbidities were dominated by diabetes in 12 cases (52.2%), arterial hypertension in 9 cases (39.1%) and dyslipidaemia in 6 cases (26.1%) (Table IV).

Table IV: Frequency of comorbidities

History	Number	Percentage (%)
Diabetes	13	56.5
Hypertension	9	39.1
Dyslipidemia	6	26.1
Chronic renal failure	5	21.7
Coronary pathology	4	17.4
Rheumatological history	3	13.0
Psychiatric disorders	3	13.0
Chronic obstructive pulmonary disease	2	8.7
Sleep apnoea syndrome	2	8.7
Pulmonary tuberculosis	2	8.7
Heart failure	2	8.7
Cardiac arrhythmia due to atrial fibrillation	2	8.7
Long-term corticosteroid therapy	2	8.7
Cerebrovascular accident	2	8.7
Anemia	2	8.7
Autoimmune disease (purpura immunological thrombocytopenic)	1	4.3

Diabetes was the main comorbidity, found in thirteen patients (56.5%), the majority of whom were type 2 (92.3%). The mean age of diabetes was 9.5 years (2- 20 years). Six patients (46.1%) were receiving oral antidiabetic drugs alone or insulin therapy alone respectively. Diabetes treatment combining oral antidiabetics and insulin was found in only one case.

None of the 23 patients had neoplastic pathology, a neurological bladder, a kidney transplant, or had received immunosuppressive treatment or chemotherapy.

Of the 5 patients with chronic renal failure, one was on haemodialysis.

6. Urological history

A urological history was reported in 9 patients (39.1%), of whom six (26.1%) had a history of renal colic due to lithiasis, and two (8.7%) had a prostate adenoma. One patient had a malformative uropathy of the pyelocal junction syndrome type. The distribution of urological histories is shown in Table V.

Table V: Breakdown of urological history

History of urology		Number	Percentage (%)
History of renal colic		6	26.1
Known urinary lithiasis		6	26.1
	caliciei	5	21.7
Site of urinary lithiasis	pyclic	1	4.3
	lumbar	2	8.7
Malformative uropathy		1	4.3

7. Risk factors for BRC carriage
7.1. Previous hospitalisation in the last 6 months

Previous hospitalisation was noted in 18 cases (78.3%). Sixteen patients (69.6%) were hospitalised in the same hospital.

The number of previous hospitalisations per patient in the last 6 months varied from 1 to 2. Six patients (13.0%) had been hospitalised 2 times in the last 6 months.

The average length of hospital stay was 17 +/- 13.6 days, with extremes ranging from 2 to 50 days.

The main departments in which patients had been hospitalised in the last 6 months were the urology department and the medical intensive care unit in 6 cases (26.1%) and 3 cases (13.0%) respectively (Table VI).

Table VI: Breakdown of patients by hospital ward in the last six months

Service	Number of cases	Percentage (%)
Urology	6	33.3
Medical resuscitation	3	16.7
Nephrology	2	11.1
Infectious diseases	1	5.6
Neurology	1	5.6
Pneumology	1	5.6
General surgery	1	5.6
Neurosurgery	1	5.6
Regional hospital	1	5.6
Private clinic	1	5.6
Total	**18**	**100**

7.2. Previous surgery in the last six months

Six patients (26.1%) had undergone surgery in the last six months.

These were urological procedures such as JJ catheter insertion in 3 cases (13%), endoscopic resection of a prostate adenoma, cholecystectomy and neurosurgery in one case (4.3%) respectively.

7.3. Previous use of antibiotics in the last six months

Antibiotic use in the six months preceding the ERC urinary tract infection was noted in 20 patients (87.0%).

The average number of antibiotics used per patient was 1.95 molecules (1 - 5 molecules).

The average total duration of antibiotic treatment received in the last six months was 10.8 +/- 2.9 days (4-15 days).

Good compliance with antibiotic treatment was noted in 18 cases (90%).

The main families of antibiotics used were beta-lactams, followed by fluoroquinolones. They were introduced in 20 cases (87.0%) and 9 cases (39.1%) respectively (Figure 10).

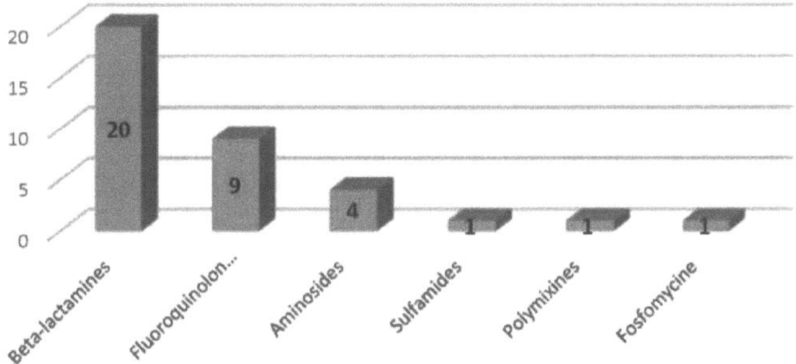

Figure 10: Frequency of use of different families of antibiotics

The types of antibiotic most frequently used were : Imipenem, amoxicillin-clavulanic acid, cefotaxime and ciprofloxacin in 6 cases (26.1%) respectively (Table VII).

Table VII: Different types of antibiotics used

Antibiotic	Number	Percentage (%)
Amoxicillin-clavulanic acid	6	26.1
Cefotaxime	6	26.1
Imipenem	6	26.1
Ciprofloxacin	6	26.1
Ertapenem	5	21.7
Gentamicin	2	8.7
Amikacin	2	8.7
Amoxicillin	1	4.3
Piperacillin-tazobactam	1	4.3
Cefexime	1	4.3
Ofloxacin	1	4.3
Levofloxacin	1	4.3
Cotrimoxazole	1	4.3
Fosfomycin	1	4.3
Colistin	1	4.3

7.4. Invasive procedure in the last six months

Fifteen patients (65.2%) had required an invasive procedure in the previous six months. These included bladder catheterisation in 15 cases, JJ catheter insertion in 3 cases (13%) and central venous catheterisation in two cases (8.7%). The distribution of the types of bladder catheterisation is detailed in Table VIII.

Table VIII: Breakdown of types of bladder catheterisation in the last 6 months

Type of bladder catheterisation	Number	Percentage (%)
Transitory	13	56.5

Intermittent	1	4.3
A demeure	1	4.3
Total	15	65.2

7.5. History of urinary tract infection

A history of urinary tract infection in the previous year was noted in 13 patients (56.5%), all of whom had required at least one hospitalisation. 6 patients (26.1%) had had more than one episode of urinary tract infection: 2 and 3 episodes in 3 cases (13.0%) respectively. Acute pyelonephritis and male urinary tract infection occurred in 8 (61.5%) and 5 (38.5%) cases respectively. A complication occurred in 6 cases (26.1%). These were acute renal failure in 4 cases (66.7%) and septic DME in 2 cases (33.3%).

The main germs isolated were *Klebsiella pneumoniae* in 9/22 cases (40.9%), *Escherichia coli* in 7/22 cases (31.8%), *Enterobacter cloacae* in 3/22 cases (13.6%) and *Enterococcus faecalis* in a single case (4.5%).

These germs were the same as those isolated during the index episode in 11/22 cases (50%).

The average length of hospital stay for these infectious episodes was 12.6 days, with extremes ranging from 7 to 17 days.

The mean time between the last history of urinary tract infection and the episode of ERC infection was 54.1 days (13 - 180 days).

7.6. History of infection other than urinary tract infection in the last six months

A history of infection other than urinary tract infection was noted in 4 cases (17.4%). These were COPD exacerbation in 2 cases, pneumonia and pulmonary tuberculosis in one case respectively. Antibiotic therapy was instituted in hospital in three patients. Apart from anti-tuberculosis drugs, the antibiotics received were : Penicillin A in 3 cases, 3rd generation cephalosporins, fluoroquinolones and aminoglycosides in one case each.

7.7. Recent trip

Recent travel was noted in two patients (8.7%). One patient had been to Saudi Arabia and the other to Algeria.

The duration of the stay abroad was 5 and 15 days respectively. There was no evidence of antibiotic treatment or hospitalisation during the stay in these countries.

In total, risk factors for complications of urinary tract infection were present in 10 patients (43.5%). These were lithiasis in 6 cases (26.1%), prostate adenoma with post-micturition residual in 2 cases (8.7%), malformative uropathy and end-stage renal disease in one case (4.3%) respectively (Figure 11).

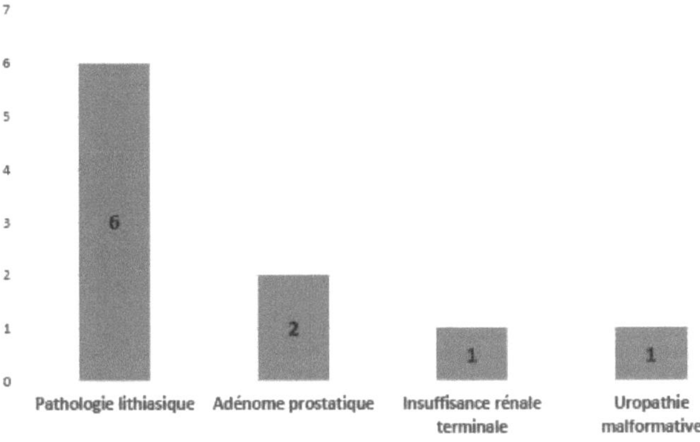

Figure 11: Distribution of complication risk factors for UTIs

At least one risk factor for ERC carriage was present in 22 patients (95.7%). These were dominated by antibiotic use in the last 6 months (87%) and hospitalisation in the last 6 months (78.3%). The distribution of the different ERC risk factors is shown in Figure 12.

The average number of DRFs for ERC carriage per patient was 3.3 +/- 1.6 (0-6).

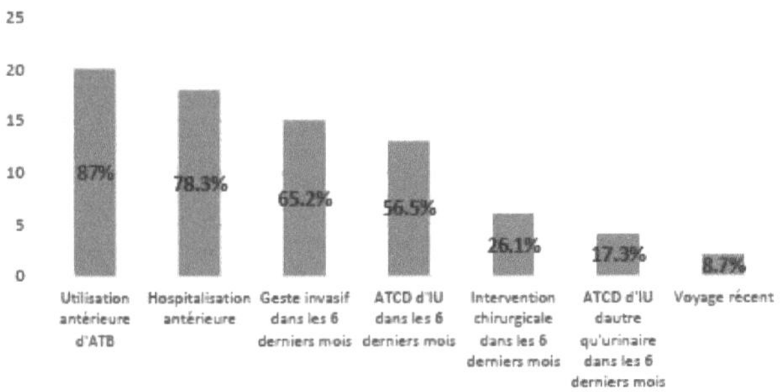

Figure 12: Breakdown of ERC risk factors

II. Clinical data

1. Functional signs

J Urinary signs :

Urinary signs were present in 9 patients (39.1%). These were urinary burning in all 9 cases, urinary frequency in 5 cases (21.7%), urinary urgency in 2 cases (8.7%) and dysuria in 4 cases (17.4%) (Figure 13).

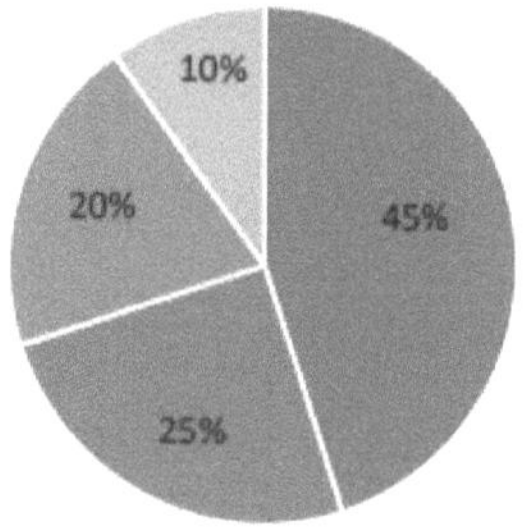

Urinary burning ■ Pollakiuria ■ Dysuria ■ Urinary urgency

Figure 13: Distribution of urinary signs

S Lower back pain :

Low back pain was present in only 3 cases (13.0%). It was unilateral in 2 cases.

S General signs :

General condition was impaired in 16 cases (69.6%).

Unquantified fever was reported in 4 cases (17.4%).

J Other associated signs :

Disturbances of consciousness were reported in 13 cases (56.5%). Respiratory signs were present in 5 cases (21.7%). These were dyspnoea in 5 cases and cough in 2 cases (8.7%).

2. Physical signs

S Signs of seriousness

- Haemodynamic parameters

Systolic blood pressure averaged 116.3 +/- 25.3 mm Hg [60-160 mm Hg]. Diastolic blood pressure averaged 66.1+/15.4 mm Hg [30-90 mm Hg]. Arterial hypotension was observed in 4 cases (17.4%).

The mean heart rate was 101.9 +/- 21.8 bpm [140- 68 bpm]. Tachycardia was found in 15 cases (65.2%). Bradycardia was not noted in any case.

- Respiratory frequency (RF)

The mean RF was 24.6 +/- 8.1 cycles/min [14- 50 cycles/min]. Polypnoea was observed in 16 cases (69.6%).

- Glasgow score (GCS):

The state of consciousness was altered in 14 cases (60.9%). Seven patients (30.4%) were comatose. The mean GCS was 10.7 with extremes ranging from 3 to 15.

- qSOFA score

The mean qSOFA score was 1.5 +/- 1.1 [0-3]. A qSOFA score $\geq$ 2 was found in

14 cases (60.9%).

- Cold extremities

Cold extremities were observed in 3 patients (13.0%).

S Fever

Fever was observed in 18 cases (78.3%). The mean temperature was 38.3 +/-
0.8°C [36.7- 39.8° C]. It was high (≥ 39° C) in 7 cases (30.4%). There was no
evidence of hypothermia.

J Lumbar shaking pain

Pain on lumbar shaking was observed in 6 cases (26.1%). It was bilateral in 2
cases.

J Rectal examination

A digital rectal examination (DRE) was performed in only 5 of the 10 men. It
was normal in 4 cases and found an enlarged, painless prostate in only one case,
ruling out the diagnosis of prostatitis.

J Gynaecological examination

In the women, the gynaecological examination found no vulvovaginitis.

J Others

Lung auscultation abnormalities were observed in 13 cases (56.5%). These were
crackling and/or snoring rales in 10 cases (43.5%) and a reduction or abolition
of vesicular murmur in 3 cases (13.0%). The auscultated rales were related to
haemodynamic PAO in 2 cases, secondary localisation of sepsis in one case and
underlying respiratory pathology in the other cases.

Cardiac auscultation was normal in 22 cases and revealed a galloping sound in
only one.

Signs of right heart failure (oedema of the lower limbs, turgidity of the jugular
veins) were present in 3 cases (13.0%).

The physical examination did not reveal any other portal of entry or other
abnormalities.

The distribution of the various physical examination anomalies is detailed in
table IX.

Table IX: Breakdown of different physical Texamen anomalies

Physical signs	Number	%
Hypotension	4	17,4
Consciousness disorders	14	60.9
q SOFA≥2	14	60,9
Cold ends	3	13.0
Fever	18	78,3
Tachycardia	15	65 ,2
Polypnoea	16	69,6
Lumbar shaking pain	6	26,1

111.Biological data

1. Cytobacteriological examination of urine

1.1. Leukocyturia

Significant leukocyturia ($>10/mm^3$) was observed in 22 cases (95.7%). The mean leukocyturia was 395.2 (1 to 1200/mm3). It was $> 150/mm3$ in 14 cases (60.9%).

1.2. Haematuria

Haematuria was observed in 14 cases (60.9%). The mean number of red blood cells per mm3 of$_{ur}$ ine was 79.1 (1 to 700/mm3).

1.3. Bacteriuria

1.3.1.Isolated bacteria

Uraculture isolated *Klebsiella pneumoniae* in 16 cases (69.6%), *Enterobacter cloacae* in 6 cases (26.1%) and *Enterobacter aerogenes* in a single case (Figure 14).

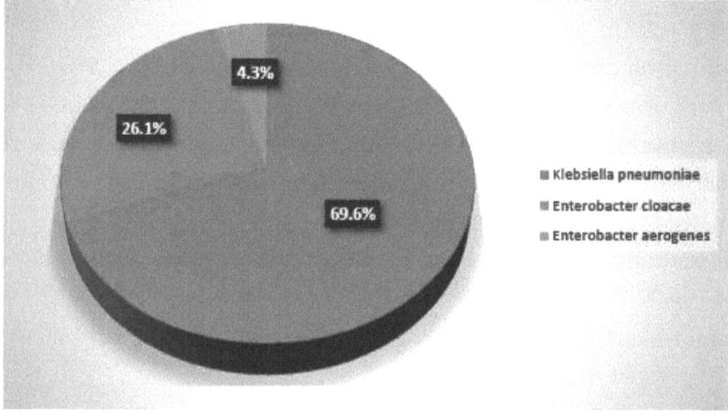

Klebsiella pneumoniae

Enterobacter cloacae

Enterobacter aerogenes

Figure 14: Frequency of different bacteria isolated

1.3.2.Distribution of bacteria by age

The average age of patients with *Klebsiella pneumoniae, Enterobacter cloacae and Enterobacter aerogenes* UTIs was 57.1, 55.8 and 69 years respectively.

The 56-65 age group was most affected by carbapenem-resistant *Klebsiella pneumoniae* urinary tract infections (50% of cases).

There was no predominant age group for carbapenem-resistant *Enterobacter* urinary tract infections (Figure 15).

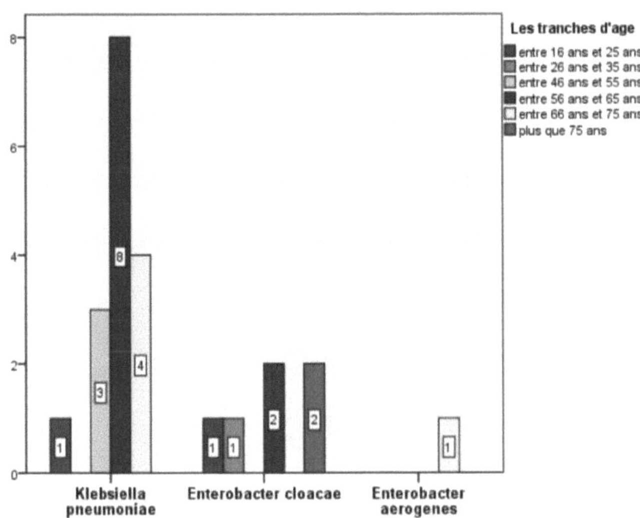

Figure 15: Breakdown of bacteria isolated by age group

1.3.3. Breakdown of bacteria by sex

There was a slight female predominance (56.2%) of carbapenem-resistant *Klebsiella pneumoniae* UTIs. Only one female patient had a urinary tract infection with *Enterobacter aerogenes, while Enterobacter cloacae* was isolated equally in both sexes (Figure 16).

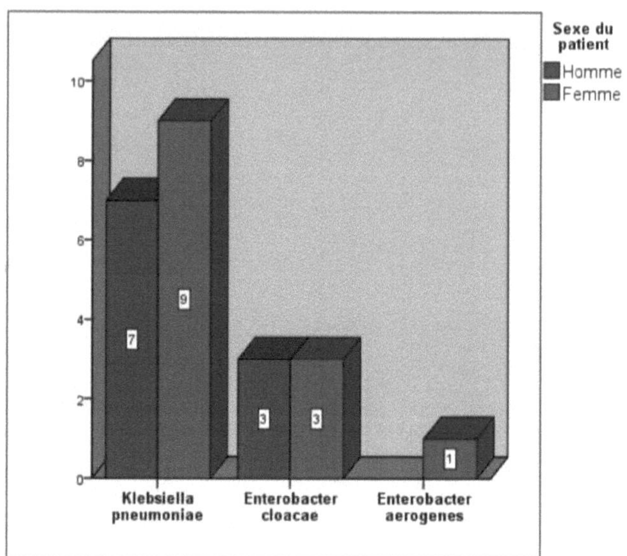

Figure 16: Breakdown of bacteria isolated by sex

1.3.4. Distribution of bacteria by type of urinary tract infection

These were mainly acute pyelonephritis and a male urinary tract infection for *K. pneumoniae*.

The distribution of bacteria according to the type of urinary infection: acute cystitis, acute pyelonephritis or UTI is summarised in Table X.

Table X: Distribution of bacteria by type of urinary tract infection

	Acute cystitis	Acute pyelonephritis	IUM	Total
Klebsiella pneumoniae	1	8	7	16
Enterobacter cloacae	0	3	3	6
Enterobacter aerogenes	0	1	0	1
Total	1	12	10	23

1.3.5. Distribution of bacteria according to the origin of the UTI: community-acquired or healthcare-associated

The urinary tract infection was community-acquired in 10 cases (43.5%) and healthcare-associated in 13 cases (56.5%). Their distribution according to the bacterium involved is shown in table XI.

Table XI: Distribution of bacteria according to the origin of UTI: (community or healthcare-associated)

	Community UI	Healthcare-associated UTI	Total
Klebsiella pneumoniae	8	8	16
Enterobacter cloacae	2	4	6

Enterobacter aerogenes	0	11
Total	10	1323

1.3.6. Distribution of bacteria by month and year

Over the four years of the study (2015-2018), the following distribution of germs was observed in descending order: _Klebsiella pneumoniae_ in first place, followed by _Enterobacter cloacae_ and _Enterobacter aerogenes_.

The frequency of _Klebsiella pneumoniae_ isolation peaked in 2015 (43.7%) (Figure 17).

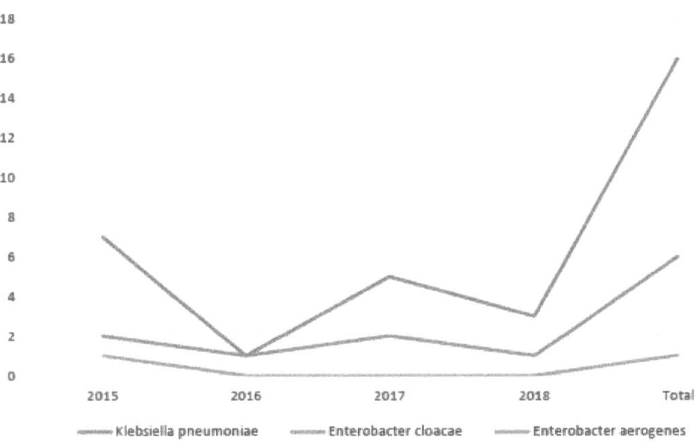

**Figure 17: Distribution of bacteria by year of isolation**

There was a clear winter-spring predominance in the isolation of these bacteria (65.2%). _Klebsiella pneumoniae_ was mainly isolated in spring (43.7%) (Figure 18).

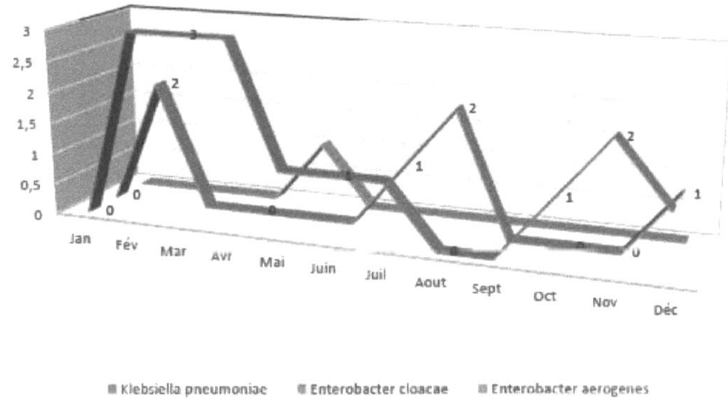

**Figure 18: Distribution of bacteria by month of isolation**

1.3.7. Breakdown of bacteria by department

The majority (47.8%) of carbapenem-resistant uropathogenic Enterobacteriaceae were isolated from patients hospitalised in the medical intensive care unit (Table XII).

The 3 strains isolated: *Klebsiella pneumoniae, Enterobacter cloacae* and *Enterobacter aerogenes* came from intensive care units in 56.2%, 66.7% and 100% of cases respectively.

Table XII: Breakdown of bacteria isolated by department of origin

	Medical resuscitation	Urology	Resuscitation anaesthesia	Infectious diseases	Pneumology	Emergencies	Total
Klebsiella pneumoniae	7	4	2	1	1	1	16
Enterobacter cloacae	3	2	1	0	0	0	6
Enterobacter aerogenes	1	0	0	0	0	0	1
Total	11	6	3	1	1	1	23

1.3.8. Susceptibility profile of isolated bacteria

The bacteria isolated were sensitive to colistin in all cases. Their sensitivity to Tamikacin and fosfomycin was partially preserved in 20 cases (87%). The sensitivity of these strains was lower to tigecycline (56.5%), cotrimoxazole (17.4%) and gentamicin (13.0%) (Table XIII).

All the strains isolated were resistant to nitrofurans.

Table XIII: Susceptibility profile of bacteria isolated

	Sensitivity to colistin (%)	Sensitivity to fosfomycin (%)	Sensitivity to Tamikacin (%)	Sensitivity to tigecycline (%)	Sensitivity to cotrimoxazole (%)	Gentamicin sensitivity (%)
Klebsiella pneumoniae	100	81.2	81.2	56.2	18.7	12.5
Enterobacter cloacae	100	100	100	50	16.7	16.7
Enterobacter aerogenes	100	100	100	100	0	0
Total	100	87	87	56.5	17.4	13.0

1.3.8.1. Susceptibility profile of *Klebsiella pneumoniae*

Klebsiella pneumoniae was sensitive to colistin in all cases. It was less sensitive to tamikacin and fosfomycin (81.2%), to tigecycline (56.2%) and to sulfonamide/trimethoprim (18.7%). It was resistant to gentamicin in 14 cases (87.5%).

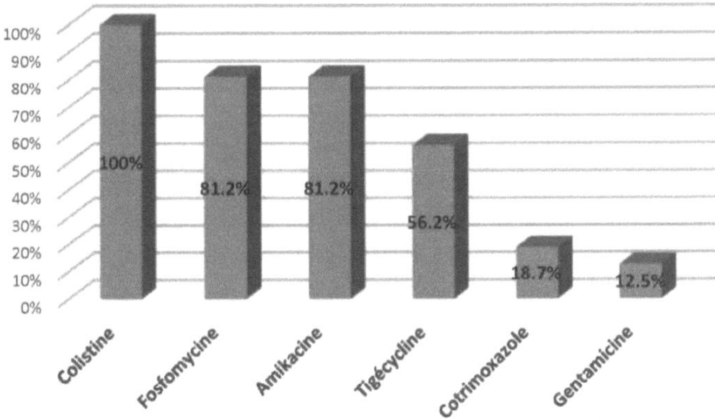

Figure 19: Susceptibility profile of Klebsiella pneumoniae to antibiotics

1.3.8.2.   Susceptibility profile of *Enterobacter cloacae*

Enterobacter cloacae was sensitive: in all cases (100%) to colistin, tamikacin and fosfomycin, in 3 cases (50%) to tigecycline and in only one case (16.7%) to sulfa/trimethoprim and gentamicin.

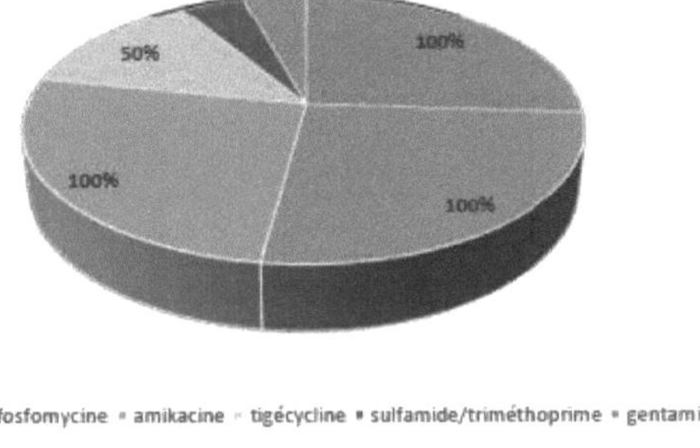

Figure 20: Susceptibility profile of Enterobacter cloacae to antibiotics

1.3.8.3.   *Enterobacter aerogenes* susceptibility profile

The only *Enterobacter aerogenes* strain isolated was sensitive to colistin, fosfomycin, tigecycline and tamikacin.

2. Other microbiological tests

2.1. Blood cultures

Blood cultures were taken in 9 patients (39.1%) with a severe form of the disease. They were contaminated and negative in 4/17 samples and positive in 7/17 samples. They had isolated the same bacteria with the same sensitivity profile as those isolated in TECBU in 4 cases. These were *Klebsiella pneumoniae*. In the other three cases, the blood culture isolated high-level

29

penicillinase-secreting *Klebsiella pneumoniae*, *Acinetobacter baumannii* and a non-groupable streptococcus.

2.2. Other bacteriological samples

A pus sample was taken in two cases. Its culture isolated the same bacteria (*Klebsiella pneumoniae*), with the same sensitivity profile, in the urine in one case and was contaminated in the other.

No bladder catheter tip culture was performed during these infectious episodes.

3. Blood count

Blood cell counts were performed in all patients, showing hyperleukocytosis in 19 cases, leukopenia in one case, thrombocytopenia in 2 cases and anaemia in 19 cases (Figure 21).

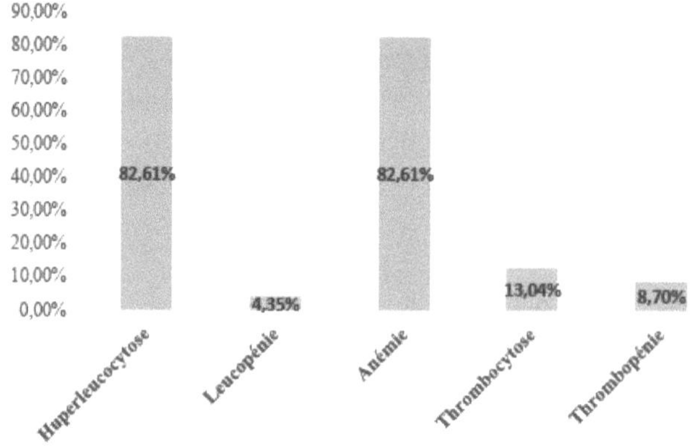

Figure 21: Distribution of haemogram abnormalities

4. C-Reactive Protein

CRP was ≥ 50 mg/l in 16 patients (69.6%). The mean level was 99.04 mg/l (3.6 - 283.4 mg/l). In complicated forms of sepsis, the mean CRP level was 128.0 mg/l [3.6 - 285.6 mg/l].

5. Blood creatinine

Mean creatinine clearance was 86.08 ml/min (3.99 - 284.32 ml/min).

Renal failure (blood creatinine ≥ 120 μmol/l) was noted in 11 cases (47.8%). It was related to: sepsis in 6 cases (54.5%) and underlying nephropathy in the other cases. Of the latter, one patient was at the haemodialysis stage.

6. Liver check-up

Hepatic cytolysis was noted in 8 cases (34.8%). It was moderate in 6 cases and > 10 times normal in two cases.

Total hyper bilirubinemia was objectified in two cases: at 71 and 188 μmol/l respectively.

7. Blood gases

Arterial gasometry was performed in 16 cases (69.6%). It revealed respiratory alkalosis in 3 cases (13.0%), hypoxaemia in one case (4.3%), metabolic acidosis in 7 cases (30.4%) and lactataemia ($\geq$ 2 mmol/l) in 9 cases (39.1%) (Figure 22).

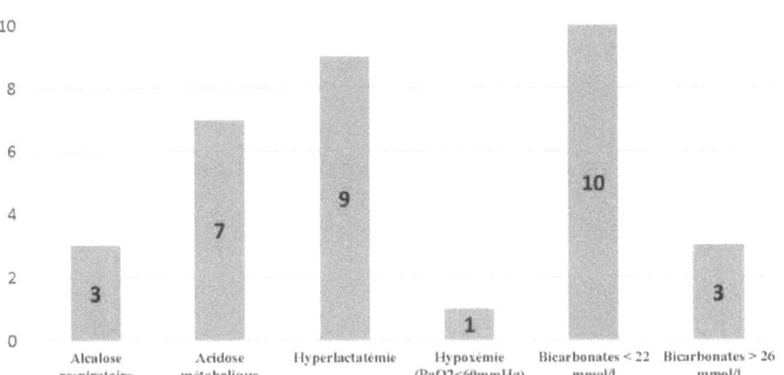

Figure 22: Distribution of arterial blood gas anomalies

8. Blood glucose

Mean blood glucose during the infectious episode was 8.82 +/- 4.36 mmol/l (3.94 - 21.08 mmol/l).

A blood glucose level $\geq$ 2.5 g/l ($\geq$ 13.75 mmol/l) was noted in 3 diabetic patients.

9. Haemostasis test (prothrombin rate, partial thromboplastin time, etc.)

Haemostasis tests were performed in 87% of cases. The mean prothrombin level was 73.3% (10 - 100%). Abnormalities in this work-up (PT < 70% and/or prolonged TCK and/or fibrinogen level > 4g/l) were observed in 6 cases (30%).

At the end of this clinico-biological assessment, the average initial SOFA score was 4.3. A SOFA score $\geq$ 2 was noted in 16 cases (Table XIV).

In all, the UTI was complicated by sepsis and septic shock in 8 cases (34.8%) respectively.

Table XIV: Breakdown of sepsis cases by gender and germ

	Women	Men	Total
Klebsiella pneumoniae	6	5	11
Enterobacter cloacae	2	2	4
Enterobacter aerogenes	1	0	1
Total	9	7	16

IV. Radiological data

1. Unprepared Urinary Tract Swab (UUTS)

AUSP was performed in 6 cases (26.1%). Calculi were found in 3 cases: lumbar calculi in 2 cases and pyelic calculi in one case.

2. Renal and bladder/vesicoprostatic ultrasound

Renal and bladder ultrasound was performed in 18 cases (78.3%). It was pathological in 6 cases (33.3%).

Ultrasound abnormalities were dominated by nephromegaly in 5 cases and dilatation of the pyelocecal cavities in 4 cases (Figure 19).

Lithiasis was detected on renal ultrasound in 3 cases: two were lumbar and one was calcific.

Ultrasonography of the prostate was performed in 4 men (40%). It was pathological in only one case, showing an enlarged prostate (Figure 23).

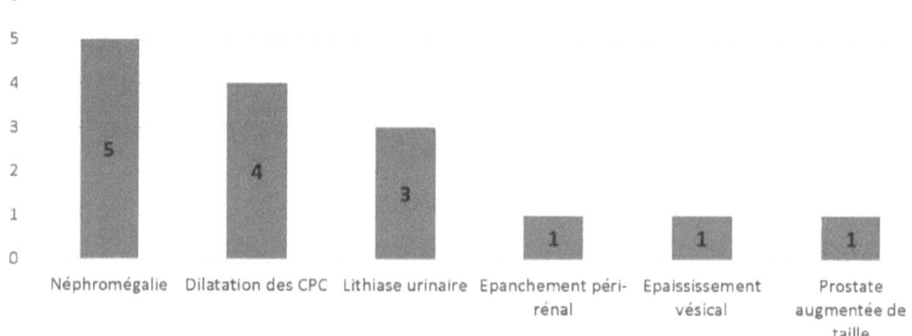

Figure 23: Ultrasound anomalies encountered

3. Uro-scanner

Uroscans were performed in 3 cases, revealing cortical thinning in 3 cases, dilatation of the pyelo-caliceal cavities and lithiasis in two cases.

4. Chest X-ray

A radiothorax was performed in all cases. It was pathological in 14 cases (60.9%). There was a well-systematised pulmonary focus in 3 cases: in relation to a secondary location of sepsis, a pneumopathy acquired under mechanical ventilation and pulmonary tuberculosis in one case each, and radiological abnormalities in relation to an underlying respiratory or cardiac pathology.

At the end of this clinical, biological and radiological assessment, the diagnosis retained was :

Acute pyelonephritis in 12 cases (52.2%), acute cystitis in one case (4.3%) and male urinary tract infection in 10 cases (43.5%) (Figure 24).

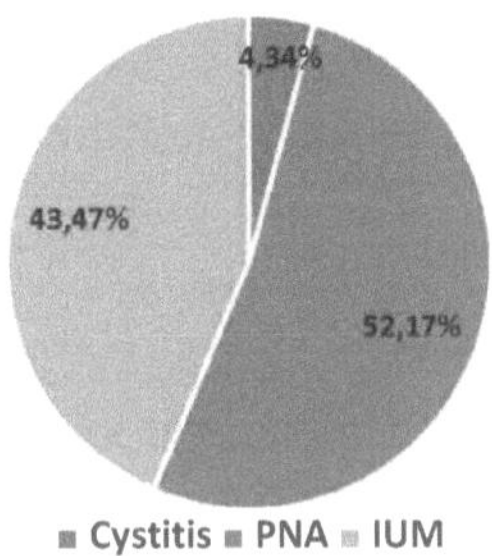

Figure 24: Distribution of clinical forms

These urinary tract infections were considered to be healthcare-associated in 13 cases (56.5%) and community-acquired in 10 cases (43.5%).

They were severe in 16 cases (69.6%). They were complicated by sepsis and septic DME in 8 cases respectively. Secondary localization occurred in only one case. This was a secondary pulmonary location.

V. Therapeutic data

1. Antibiotic therapy

Antibiotic treatment was prescribed in 22 cases (95.7%). One patient died before receiving antibiotics due to a delay in diagnosis.

The mean time from onset of clinical signs to initiation of active antibiotic therapy was 5.6 +/- 3.2 days (2- 12 days). It was $\geq$ 3 days in 68.2% of cases.

1.1. Molecules used

The main drugs prescribed as first-line treatment were tamikacin, tigecycline and colimycin in 15 cases (68.2%), 11 cases (50%) and 10 cases (45.5%) respectively (Table XV).

Table XV: Different antibiotics prescribed as first-line treatment

Antibiotic	Number of cases	Percentage (%)
Amikacin	15	68.2
Tigecycline	11	50.0
Colimycin	10	45.5
Imipenem	6	27.3
Fosfomycin	5	22.7
Tazocillin	2	9.1
Ciprofloxacin	2	9.1
Cotrimoxazole	1	4.5
Ertapenem	1	4.5
Ceftazidime	1	4.5

Adjustment of the initial antibiotic therapy to the antibiogram data was necessary in 9 cases (40.9%). The average switchover time was 6.1 days (2 - 12 days). All cases were escalated.

The main antibiotics prescribed for the treatment of these documented ERC urinary tract infections were: Tamikacin and tigecy cline in 15 cases (68.2%) and 11 cases (50.0%) respectively. The distribution of antibiotics prescribed after adjustment for antibiogram data is shown in Table XVI.

Table XVI: Antibiotics prescribed after bacteriological documentation

Active antibiotic	Number	Percentage (%)
Amikacin	15	68.2
Tigecycline	11	50
Colistin	10	45.5
Fosfomycin	5	22.7
Cotrimoxazole	1	4.5

1.2. Monotherapy or combination of active antibiotics

Three patients had received monotherapy (13.6%) based on fosfomycin and tigecycline in 2 cases and 1 case respectively for the treatment of 2 acute pyelonephritis and one MUI.

A combination of active antibiotics was prescribed in 19 cases (86.4%).

Tigecycline and fosfomycin were used in combination in 10 out of 11 cases (90.9%) and 3 out of 5 cases (60%) respectively.

Amikacin and colistin were prescribed in combination with other active antibiotics.

Cotrimoxazole was prescribed in only one case. It was combined with amikacin.

A patient with *Klebsiella pneumoniae* UTI was prescribed triple antibiotic therapy with imipenem, ertapenem and amikacin.

The most frequently prescribed combinations of antibiotics were colimycin + tigecycline and tigecycline + amikacin in 5 cases (22.7%) respectively (Figure 25).

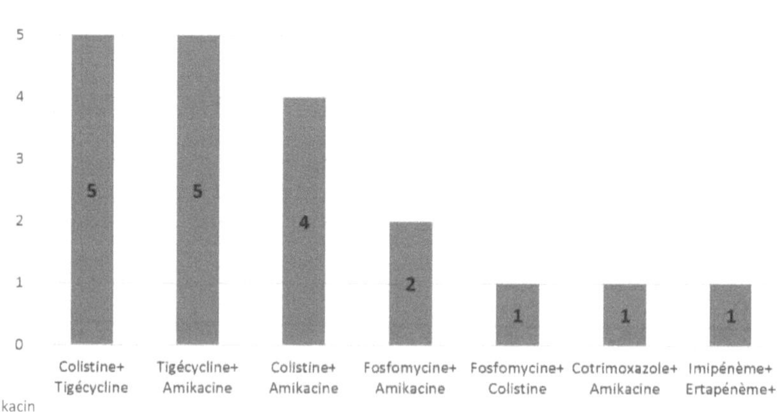

Figure 25: Combinations of active antibiotics

The mean duration of the combination was 5.2 +/- 2.2 days (3 - 10 days) with a median of 5 days.

1.3. Route of administration

All patients had received intravenous antibiotic therapy. The intramuscular route was not indicated in any case.

Only one patient with acute pyelonephritis had received oral Cotrimoxazole in combination with Tamikacin.

1.4. Duration of treatment in hospital

The average duration of in-hospital treatment after the onset of infection was 25.5 days, with a median of 15 days and extremes ranging from 4 to 100 days. More than 30 days were required in 4 cases (17.4%).

A patient with acute uncomplicated pyelonephritis caused by cotrimoxazole-sensitive *Klebsiella pneumoniae* was hospitalised for 4 days.

One patient required treatment for 100 days in connection with complications of prolonged resuscitation for a deep coma.

2. Other therapeutic measures

2.1. Invasive procedures

Some patients required invasive procedures:

- Tracheal intubation and artificial ventilation in 11 cases (47.8%)
- Placement of a central catheter in 7 cases (30.4%)
- Vascular filling/ vasoactive drugs in 16 cases (69.6%)
- Parenteral nutrition in 3 cases (13.0%)
- Haemodialysis sessions in 3 cases (13.0%).

The breakdown of invasive procedures is shown in Table XVII.

Table XVII: Breakdown of invasive procedures

Invasive procedures	Number	%
Vascular filling and/or use of vasoactive drugs	16	69.6
Tracheal intubation and mechanical ventilation	11	47.8
Tracheotomy	7	30.4
Central venous catheter	7	30.4
Parenteral nutrition	3	13.0
Haemodialysis sessions	3	13.0
JJ probe removal	1	4.3
Feeding gastrectomy	1	4.3

2.2. Isolation

Carriage of a CRB was not mentioned in any of the patient files, although it is mentioned in the care records of patients admitted to intensive care units.

Outside intensive care units, isolation was only possible in one case. This was a patient admitted to the internal medicine department with a male urinary tract infection.

VI. Evolutionary data

1. Favourable evolution

The outcome was favourable in 15 cases (65.2%) with a mean follow-up time of 486.7 days +/- 210.7 days.

1.1. Clinic

Functional signs (urinary signs and lumbar pain) and physical signs disappeared completely in 11 cases and regressed in 4 cases.

The mean time to disappearance of functional signs was 3 +/- 0.63 days (2 - 4 days).

The average time to apyrexia for febrile patients was 2.8 days (2- 4 days).

1.2. Biology

Normalization of white blood cell and platelet counts was noted in 13 and 15 cases respectively. In the majority of cases (85%), a fall in CRP was observed more than 72 hours after the start of antibiotic therapy, adapted to the antibiogram data.

Among the 15 patients who progressed well, there were no cases of recurrence.

2. Unfavourable trend

2.1. Complications

A complication related to the urinary tract infection occurred in 16 cases (69.6%).

A secondary pulmonary site occurred in a patient with *Klebsiella pneumoniae* UTI complicated by septic EDC. The patient presented with hypoxaemic pneumonitis, with a well-systematised opacity in the left basal focus on chest X-ray. The patient required mechanical ventilation. The patient died.

There were no cases of renal abscess or nephritis.

Four patients (17.4%) had presented with decompensation of a condition. Diabetes decompensation occurred in 2 cases and haemodynamic PAO in 2 cardiac patients.

Six patients (26.1%) had developed a complication related to prolonged dorsal recumbency: pressure sores in 5 cases and deep vein thrombosis in one case (Table XVIII).

Table XVIII: Distribution of complications

	Complications	Number	%
Complications	Organ failure	15	65.2
infectious	Secondary septic location	1	4.3
Related	Pressure sores	5	21.7

complications			
decubitus	Deep vein thrombosis	1	4.3
Decompensation	Simple diabetic ketosis	1	4.3
a defect	Diabetic ketoacidosis	1	4.3
	Hemodynamic OAP	2	8.7

2.2. Deaths

Death occurred in seven cases (30.4%). These were refractory septic shock in 3 cases (13.0%), deep coma in 3 cases and acute respiratory failure in one case.

The mean time between the onset of symptoms of carbapenem-resistant enterobacteriaceae UTI and death was 41.1 +/- 36.5 days (4 - 100 days).

VII. Economic data

The cost of managing these ERC urinary tract infections was obtained by calculating the sum of the cost of antibiotic therapy and the cost of the hospital stay.

1. Cost of antibiotic therapy

The average cost of antibiotic treatment was 1998.2 +/- 1591.2 DT, ranging from 54.7 to 5629.2 DT.

2. Cost of hospital stay

The median cost of a hospital stay, including all expenditure on nursing care, hospital accommodation, hygiene and food, was 840 DT (140 - 6000 DT).

3. Total cost

By calculating the sum of the costs of antibiotic therapy and hospital stay, we can estimate the overall cost of managing a urinary tract infection with ERC. In fact, the average overall cost was 3334.4 DT +/- 2844.9 (234.0 - 11149.2 DT). Table XIX shows the distribution of different costs according to the type of UTI. Table XX shows the distribution of different costs according to germs.

Table XIXDistribution of costs according to type of urinary infection

	Average cost of stay (DT)	Average cost of antibiotic therapy (DT)	Overall average cost (DT)
Acute pyelonephritis	1942.3	2232.8	4175.1
Male urinary tract infection	748.0	1493.5	2241.5
Total	1345.1	1863.1	3208.3

Table XX: Distribution of different costs according to the germ involved

	Average cost of stay (DT)	Average cost of antibiotic therapy (DT)	Overall average cost (DT)
Klebsiella pneumoniae	1533.1	1768.1	3301.2
Enterobacter cloacae	1266.7	1901.5	3168.2
Enterobacter aerogenes	840.0	4263.0	5103.0
Total	1213.3	2644.2	3857.5

Table XXI: Summary table of various observations

	Age	Gender	Comorbidities	Clinical form	Severity of the clinical picture	Isolated germ	Emnirim treatment	Appropriate TBA	Time limit for treatment	Evolution	Deaths | | s| | | j
1	58	Men	Diabetes, CKD,	IUM	Severe sepsis	*K.pneumoniae*	Ceñazidime+ CiDrofloxacin	Fosfomycin+ Amikacin	6j	Favourable	no
2	58	Woman	-	NAP	-	*K.pneumoniae*	-	Colimycin+ Fosfomvcine	Zi	Favourable	no
3	56	Woman	Diabetes, hypertension, dyslipidaemia, DDB, TT? C¹	Cystitis	-	*K.pneumoniae*	-	Colimycin+ Amikacin	IOj	Favourable	no
4	56	Men	Diabetes, coronary	IUM	-	*K.pneumoniae*	-	Colimycin+ Tiumecvcline	6J	Favourable	no
5	62	Woman	Diabetes, Dvslinidemia	NAP	-	*E. cloacae*	-	Fosfomycin+ Amikacin	8j	Favourable	no
6	80	Men	-	IUM	-	*E. cloacae*	-	Fosfomycin	Sj	Unfavourable	-
7	73	Men	Diabetes	IUM	Severe sepsis	*K pneumoniae*	-	Tigecycline+ Amikacin	4j	Favourable	no
8	47	Men	Diabetes	IUM	Severe sepsis	*K pneumoniae*	-	Colimycin+ Amikacin	3j	Favourable	no
9	60	Woman	Diabetes, hypertension, CKD	NAP	Severe sepsis	*K pneumoniae*	-	Colimycin+ Amikacin	2j	Favourable	no
10	80	Men	Diabetes, hypertension, COPD	IUM	EDC septic	*E. cloacae*	Tazocillin+ CiDrofloxacin	Colimycin+ Amikacin	4j	Favourable	no
11	69	Woman	Diabetes, Hypertension, HvDothvroidism	NAP	EDC septic	*E. aerogenes*	Tazocillin+ Amikacin	Colimycin+ Tisecvcline	IOj	Unfavourable to D 18	
12	62	Woman	Diabetes, hypertension, dyslipidemia,	NAP	Severe sepsis	*K pneumoniae*	Imipenem+ Amikacin	Tigecycline	3j	Favourable	no
13	30	Woman	-	NAP	Severe sepsis	*E. cloacae*	Imipenem	Tigecycline+ Amikacin	Zi	Favourable	no
14	60	Woman	Gonarthrosis	NAP	Severe sepsis	*K pneumoniae*	Imipenem	Colimycin+ Tisecvcline	IOj	Favourable	no
15	65	Men	COPD	IUM	EDC septic	*E. cloacae*	-	Tigecycline+ Amikacin	3j	Favourable	no
16	57	Woman	Diabetes, hypertension, dyslipid½nie, *stroke*	NAP	EDC septic	*K pneumoniae*	-	Tigecycline+ Amiklin	6j	Favourable	to J73
17	48	Men	.	IUM	Severe sepsis	*K pneumoniae*	-	Colimycin+ Tisecvcline	3j	Unfavourable at D58	
18	18	Woman	-	NAP	EDC septic	*E. cloacae*	-	Tigecycline+ Amikacin	3j	Unfavourable at D60	
19	75	Men	Hypertension, IiVDODhvsar adenoma	IUM	EDC septic	*K pneumoniae*	Imipenem+ Colimvcine	Colimycin+ Tisecvcline	9j	Unfavourable at D20	
20	18	Woman	-	NAP	EDC septic	*K pneumoniae*	Imipenem+ Amiklin	Fosfomycin	12	Unfavourable at J91	
21	68	Woman	Diabetes, hypertension, SAS	NAP	EDC septic	*K pneumoniae*	-	-	-	Unfavourable to J4	
22	46	Men	Consenital encephalopathy	IUM	-	*K pneumoniae*	-	Imipenem+ Ertapenem+	3j	Favourable	no
23	73	Woman	Diabetes, hypertension, CKD, coronary heart disease	NAP	-	*K pneumoniae*	-	Cotrimoxazole + Amikacin	2j	Favourable	no

VIII. Analytical study

A univariate analysis of the different risk factors according to the type of CRB isolated showed an association between bladder catheterisation and carbapenem-resistant *Klebsiella pneumoniae* urinary tract infection (*p*= 0.026) (Table XXII). There was a non-significant association between the isolation of this bacterium and the presence of a history of urinary tract infection *(p=0.092)*.

Table XXII: Relationship between risk factors for acquiring ERC urinary tract infections and the type of germ isolated

	Klebsiella pneumoniae N	*p*	*Enterobacter cloacae* N (%)	*p*

	(%)			
Gender :				
-Female	9 (69.2)		3(23.1)	
-Male	7 (70)	0.663	4(30.0)	0.537
Age :				
- ≥65 years	4 (50.0)		3(37.5)	
- < 65 years	12 (80.0)	0.156	3(20.0)	0.336
Diabetes :				
-yes	10 (76.9)		2 (15.4)	
_- no_	6 (60.0)	0.337	4 (40.0)	0.197
HTA				
-yes	7 (77.8)		1 (11.1)	
_-no_	9 (64.3)	0.418	5 (35.7)	0.208
Dyslipidemia				
-yes	5 (83.3)		1 (16.7)	
_-no_	11 (64.7)	0.382	5 (29.4)	0.490
COPD				
-yes	1 (50.0)		1 (50.0)	
_-no_	15 (71.4)	0.526	5 (23.8)	0.462
Chronic renal failure				
-yes	5(100)		0 (0.0)	
_-no_	18 (61.1)	0.130	6 (18)	-
Haemodialysis				
-yes	1 (100)		0 (0.0)	
_-no_	15 (68.2)	0.696	6 (27.3)	-
Long-term corticosteroid therapy				
-yes	2(100)		0 (0.0)	
_-no_	14 (66.7)	0.474	6 (28.6)	-
Urinary lithiasis				
-yes	5 (83.3)		1 (16.7)	
_-no_	11 (64.7)	0.382	5 (29.4)	0.490
Urinary catheterisation				
-yes	13 (86.7)		2 (13.3)	
_-no_	3 (37.5)	0.026	4 (50.0)	0.087
History of urinary tract infection				
-yes	11 (84.6)		2 (15.4)	
_-no_	5 (50.0)	0.092	4 (40.0)	0.197
History of hospitalisation in the last 6 months				
-yes	14 (77.8)		4(22.2)	
_-no_	2 (40.0)	0.142	2(40.0)	0.392
History of antibiotic use in the last 6 months				
-yes	15 (75.0)		5 (25.0)	
_-no_	1 (50.0)	0.481	0 (0.0)	-
History of surgery in the last 6 months				
-yes	4(66.7)		2 (33.3)	
_-no_	12(70.6)	0.618	4 (23.5)	0.510

The clinical, biological and evolutionary characteristics, depending on the germ isolated, are summarised in Table XXIII :

Table XXIII: Relationship between the various clinical, biological and evolutionary features of ERC UTIs and the type of germ isolated

	Klebsiella pneumoniae N (%)	Enterobacter cloacae N (%)	p
Clinical elements			
Clinical form			
- ANP	8 (53.3)	3 (50.0)	
- IUM	7 (46.7)	3 (50.0)	0.633
Fever	13 (81.3)	5 (83.3)	0.708
Urinary signs	7 (77.8)	2 (100)	0.655
Lumbar shaking pain	4 (44.4)	2 (66.7)	0.500
Severe sepsis	7 (43.8)	1 (16.7)	0.255
EDC septic	4 (25.0)	3 (50.0)	0.267
Biological elements			
Leukocyturia	15 (93.8)	6 (100)	0.727
Hyperleukocytosis	12 (75.0)	6 (100)	0.249
CRP> 50mg/dl	12 (75.0)	3 (50.0)	0.267
Hyperlactatemia	5 (62.5)	3 (100)	0.339
Hypoxia	1 (11.1)	2 (50.0)	0.203
Evolving elements			
Hospital stay > 15 days	7 (43.8)	2 (33.3)	0.523
Time to apyrexia ≥ 3 days	5 (71.4)	2 (66.7)	0.708
Complications	11 (68.8)	4 (66.7)	0.651
Deaths	5 (31.6)	1 (16.7)	0.459
Total cost > 2000 DT	8 (50.0)	4 (66.7)	0.417

Analysis of these data shows no difference in clinical, biological, evolutionary or financial terms between *K pneumoniae* and *Enterobacter* infections.

Analysis of the course according to the antibiotic therapy prescribed found no association between the prescription of a monotherapy and an unfavourable outcome (*p=0.7*). Prescription of tigecycline was significantly associated with an unfavourable outcome (*p=0.032*) (table XXIV).

Table XXIV relationship between antibiotic therapy prescribed and outcome

	Favourable outcome N= (%)	Unfavourable trend N= (%)	p
Monotherapy	2 (66.7)	1 (33.3)	
Combination of antibiotics	13 (68.4)	6 (31.6)	0.705
Prescribed colistin (in combination)	7 (70)	3 (30)	0.616

Tigecycline prescribed	5 (45.5)	6 (54.5)	0.032
Tigecycline monotherapy	1(100)	0 (0)	0.682
Tigecycline in combination	4 (40)	6 (60)	0.015
Fosfomycin prescribed	4 (80)	1 (20)	0.477
Fosfomycin monotherapy	1 (50)	1 (50)	0.545
Fosfomycin in combination	3(100)	0 (0)	0.295
Amikacin prescribed (in combination)	10 (76.9)	3 (23.1)	0.276
Cotrimoxazole prescribed (in combination)	1(100)	0 (0)	0.682
Imipenem prescribed (in combination)	1(100)	0 (0)	0.682
Ertapenem (in combination)	1(100)	0 (0)	0.682
Colistin+ Tigecycline	2 (40)	3 (60)	0.160
Colistin+ Amikacin	4(100)	0 (0)	0.187
Tigecycline+ amikacin	2 (40)	3 (60)	0.160
Fosfomycin+ Amikacin	2(100)	0 (0)	0.455
Fosfomycin+ Colistin	1(100)	0 (0)	0.682
Cotrimoxazole+ Amikacin	1(100)	0 (0)	0.682
Imipenem+ Ertapenem+ Amikacin	1(100)	0 (0)	0.682

Analysis of the outcome according to the various prognostic factors showed no association with age, sex, the presence of co-morbidities (diabetes and hypertension, IR), or the time taken to start appropriate antibiotic therapy. Only the presence of sepsis or EDC and admission to intensive care were associated with an unfavourable outcome.

Table XXV: Relationship between prognostic factors for ERC urinary tract infections and evolution

	Favourable trend N %)	Unfavourable trend N %)	p
Advanced age ≥ 65 years	4 (50)	4 (50)	0.253
Female sex	8 (61.5)	5 (38.5)	0.510
Presence of co-morbidities	10 (66.7)	5 (33.3)	0.596
≥3 comorbidities	6 (75)	2 (25)	0.404
Diabetes	9 (69.2)	4 (30.8)	0.490
HTA	5 (55.6)	4 (44.4)	0.367
Dyslipidemia	4 (66.7)	2 (33.3)	0.660
COPD	2 (100)	0 (0)	0.415
Chronic renal failure	4 (80)	1 (20)	0.414
CKD at haemodialysis stage	1 (100)	0 (0)	0.652
Heart failure	2 (100)	0 (0)	0.415
Autoimmune disease	0 (0)	1 (100)	0.348
Long-term corticosteroid therapy	0 (0)	2 (100)	0.111
Severe sepsis or EDC	8 (50)	8 (50)	0.026
Admission to the intensive care unit	7 (50)	7 (50)	0.069
Time between onset of clinical signs and effective antibiotic therapy ≥ 3 days	9 (75)	3 (25)	0.693

| *Inappropriate empirical antibiotic therapy* | 5 (62.5) | 3 (37.5) | 0.510 |

I.   Epidemiology   of   carbapenem-resistant Enterobacteriaceae

The emergence of ERCs around the world has become a threat to public health. It has prompted public health authorities to prioritise vigorous action to prevent these infections.

1. Worldwide

1.1. KPC-producing Enterobacteriaceae

They represent the type of carbapenemase most frequently reported worldwide among class A beta-lactamases. They have been identified mainly in *Klebsiella pneumoniae* and more rarely in other enterobacteria (*Escherichia coli, Proteus mirabilis, Enterobacter cloacae*) [24]. The first case of KPC was reported in the United States (North Carolina) in 1996 [9]. Since then, these strains have spread to several countries around the world, where they have become endemic (Greece, Italy, etc.). The reservoir of these enzymes is essentially *K. pneumoniae*, which is mainly distributed in hospitals.

1.1.1 North America

According to a systematic review of articles published between 1/1/2010 and 1/2/2016, the annual incidence of carbapenem-resistant Enterobacteriaceae in the United States ranged from 0.3 to 2.93 cases/100,000 people [25]. KPC-producing strains were the only carbapenemases identified (representing 47.9% of all ERCs) in a study of 7 US metropolitan areas [26].

Rapid dissemination of *Klebsiella pneumoniae* strains producing KPC-2 has been reported in the north-east of the country, mainly in New York [27].

The first cases of KPC variants 4, 5, 6, 8 and 10 were isolated in Puerto Rico [28].

According to the Canadian Antimicrobial Resistance Surveillance System (CARSS) report published in 2017, 2106 EPCs, 40% of which were KPC-secreting, were isolated in Canada between 2008 and 2016.

1.1.2 South America

KPC-producing bacteria have also emerged in South America.

In 2006, Colombia was the first South American country to identify a KPC-producing strain of *Pseudomonas aeroginosa*. Since then, other Latin American countries have reported the spread of KPC-producing Enterobacteriaceae, including Argentina, Chile and Brazil [29] [30].

1.1.3 Europe

In Europe, the highest incidence of KPC-secreting Enterobacteriaceae was noted in Mediterranean countries mainly in Italy and Greece. These two countries were the only European countries that reported an endemic situation for KPC in

2014- 2015 [31]. The European Bacterial Antibiotic Resistance Surveillance Centre (EARS Net) declared Greece "an epicentre" from which KPC-producing strains spread to other European countries. Indeed, the first Greek case of KPC-2 producing KP was identified in 2008 [32] and since then the number of cases has increased. Spyropoulou et al found in a Greek retrospective study (January 2005-December 2014) that 48% of *Klebsiella pneumoniae* strains isolated were carbapenemase-producing, of which 80% were KPC [33].

The first Italian case of *Klebsiella pneumoniae* producing KPC-3 was also identified in 2008 [34] and since then, this carbapenemase has spread throughout the country [35].

1.1.4 Middle East

The first epidemic of KPC-producing *Klebsiella pneumoniae* in the Middle East was described in Israel by Leavitt et al. (2004-2006) [36].

A national strategy to control the spread of ERC in Israel was launched in 2007 and has reduced the incidence of hospital-acquired ERC infections from 55.5 to 4.8 cases/100,000 patient days [37].

1.1.5 Asia

In a Chinese multicentre study conducted in 2015, KPC-producing strains represented 50.3% of all carbapenemase-secreting Enterobacteriaceae [38]. The predominant KPC-producing *Klebsiella pneumoniae* clone was ST11 in the multicentre study by Yan Qi et al [39].

1.2. MBL-producing Enterobacteriaceae

MBL-type carbapenemases (especially NDM) appear to be concentrated in Asia. The first patient in whom bla-NDM-1 was detected was a Swedish man who travelled to India in 2007 and contracted a *Klebsiella pneumoniae* urinary tract infection [10]. Since then, several studies have shown the spread of NDM-1-producing Enterobacteriaceae in India, Pakistan and Bangladesh [40] [41].

NDM-1 secreting strains have also been reported in China, but appear to be less widespread than in India [42].

In a multicentre study conducted in China in 2015, the carbapenemase most isolated from *Escherchia coli* strains was NDM (29/39 or 74.4%) [38].

In Europe, NDM-producing strains were found in Romania, Poland and Denmark. However, VIM is the predominant MBL in other European countries such as Spain, Italy and Hungary [31].

In addition, the role of contact with health facilities and the role of travel to NDM-endemic countries such as India in the emergence of these strains in European countries should be emphasised.

In North America, MBL-secreting strains are rarely isolated. An outbreak of NDM-1-producing *Klebsiella pneumoniae* was reported in 2012 in Denever

[43]. VIM and IMP carbapenemases are even rarer.

A multicentre study carried out in 7 South American countries (20122014) revealed that EPCs carried the bla VIM and bla NDM genes in 9% and 8% respectively [44].

In the run-up to the 2016 Olympic Games, the bla NDM-1 gene was identified in EPCs present in 2 famous aquatic environments in Rio de Janero (Rodrigo de Freitas Lagoon and Carioca River) [45].

1.3. OXA-48-producing Enterobacteriaceae

The worldwide spread of OXA-type carbapenemases is mainly due to the propagation of strains producing OXA-48 and, to a lesser extent, OXA-181.

The first OXA-48-producing *Klebsiella pneumoniae* was reported in Turkey in 2001 [13]. Since then, it has continued to spread throughout the country. Indeed, in 2014- 2015, Turkey represented the highest epidemiological level of OXA-48-secreting strains (stage 5 "endemic situation") [31].

These strains have rapidly emerged in the Middle East and North Africa [46] [47].

In Europe, most cases are attributed to patients imported from North Africa. The epidemiological level in 2014- 2015 was stage 4 ("inter-regional spread") for Spain, France, Belgium and Romania [31].

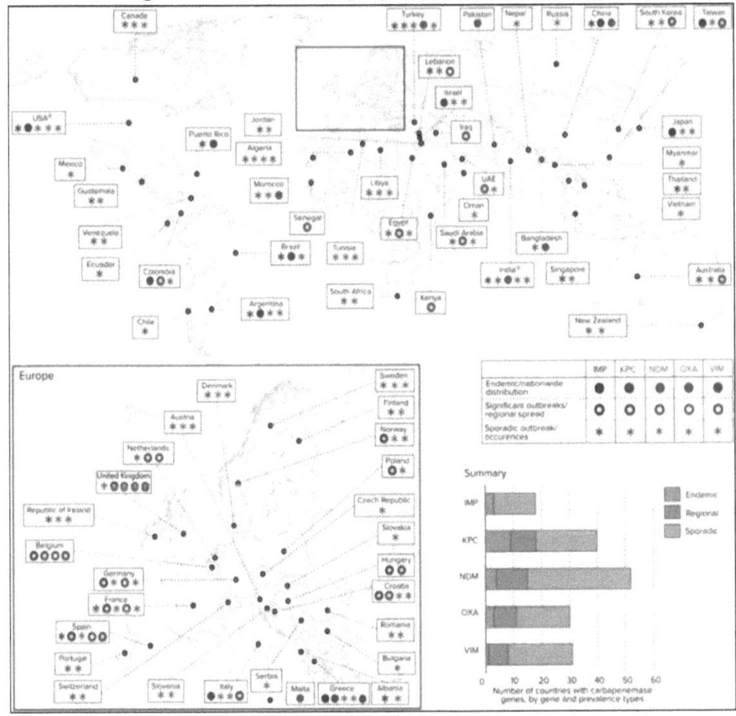

45

2. In Africa

2.1. KPC-producing Enterobacteriaceae

Few data are available on the epidemiology of KPC-producing Enterobacteriaceae in Africa.

According to a systematic review of the literature, only 3 studies, carried out in Egypt, Tanzania and South Africa, had reported the isolation of KPC-secreting Enterobacteriaceae [49].

In Egypt, 14 KPC-producing strains of *Klebsiella pneumoniae* were isolated from the Suez Canal University Hospital [50].

In a single-centre study in Tanzania, only 8 strains out of 103 EPCs were KPC-producing [51].

2.2. MBL-producing Enterobacteriaceae

In Africa, 4 metallo-beta-lactamases (NDM, VIM, IMP, DIM) have been identified in enterobacteria [49].

The first African case of NDM-1 was identified in Kenya (on the basis of EPC isolated from urine or urethral pus) in patients admitted to the wards of Aga Kham University Hospital between 2007 and 2009 [52].

NDM-producing Enterobacteriaceae (mainly *Klebsiella pneumoniae*) have mainly been identified in hospitals (intensive care units or surgical wards) in Kenya, Nigeria and South Africa [49].

IMP has only been identified in Morocco, Tunisia and Tanzania [53] [54] [55] [50]. DIM-1 has only been found in Sierra Leone [56].

In fact, only 3 studies have reported the detection of IMP-1 in Africa: two in Morocco (4 cases isolated from community urinary tract infections) [53] [54] and one in Tunisia; carried out at Kasserine hospital in 2010 and finding 10 NDM-1-producing ERC strains in the intensive care unit [54].

2.3. OXA-48-producing Enterobacteriaceae

Several studies have shown the endemicity of the OXA-48 enzyme in North African countries such as Morocco and Tunisia [49].

OXA 181-secreting strains of *Klebsiella pneumoniae* have been isolated from patients hospitalised in South Africa [57].

In a study by Leski et al carried out in Sierra Leone, carbapenemases OXA-51Like and OXA-58 were identified in EPCs [55].

3. In Tunisia

There are very few epidemiological studies describing the resistance mechanisms of enterobacteria to the carbapenems present in our country, and their geographical distribution.

Oxacillinase OXA-48 appears to be the most frequently described carbapenemase in Tunisia (Table XV).

A nosocomial outbreak of OXA-48-secreting *Providencia stuartii* was reported in the Habib Bourguiba University Hospital in Sfax in 2011 [58].

At the same hospital, 21/153 (13.7%) strains of *Klebsiella pneumoniae* isolated between 2009 and 2010 were OXA-48 secretors [59].

A single-centre study carried out at CHU Taher Sfar Mahdia (2015- 2016) showed that among 220 strains of *Klebsiella pneumoniae*; 29 (13.2%) were resistant to carbapenems of which the most frequently isolated carbapenemase was OXA-48 like (75.9%) [60].

Other OXA-48 variants, notably OXA-204, have been reported in Tunisia [61].

In 2006, a nosocomial epidemic due to a strain of *Klebsiella pneumoniae* producing a VIM-4 type metallo-enzyme occurred in Sfax [62].

In 2010, Chouchani et al found *Klebsiella pneumoniae* strains secreting VIM and IMP in rivers in Tunisia (Oued Meliane and Oued Solmane) [63].

In addition, epidemics of VIM-2-secreting *Pseudomonas aeruginosa* have been reported [64] [65].

To date, no cases of KPC-secreting enterobacteria have been reported in Tunisia.

Table XXVI: Studies of UTIs caused by carbapenemase-secreting Enterobacteriaceae in Tunisia

Year of isolation	2010	2009-10	2005	2009	2011	2010	2012	2009-11
Type of study	Case report	Sunzeillance provided by laboratories	Sunzeillance provided by laboratories	Case report	Sunzeillance provided by laboratories	Cross-sectional study	Case report	Sunzeillance provided by laboratories
Type of sample	urine	ND	Urine, blood, wound, catheter, brain abscess, sputum	Sputum or blood	Rectal, nasal, axillary, environmental swabs	environmental swabs	Sternal pus	Pus, urine, blood
Bacteria	*K.pneumoniae*	*K.pneumoniae*	*K.pneumoniae*	*K.pneumoniae*	*P. Stuartii*	*E. coli K.pneumoniae*	*K.pneumoniae*	*K.pneumoniae C.freundii*
Number of strains positive/ Total number of strains tested (%)	ND	21/153 (14)	11/11 (100)	ND	13/13 (100)	13/46 (28)	ND	ND
The carbapenemase described	ONA-48 (2)	ONA-48 (21)	VIM-4(11)	ONA-48 (1)	ONA-48 (13)	VIM-2 (4) NDM-I		ONA-48 (4) ONA-48 (1)
Community/ Nosocomial	N	N			N			N
Age	ND	ND	A	A	A	ND	A	A/F
Reference	[66]	[59]	[62]	[67]	[58]	[68]	[69]	[70]

II. Risk factors for carbapenem-resistant Enterobacteriaceae urinary tract infections

1. Age

According to a review of the literature covering articles published from 1966 to 2016 and studying the risk factors for multidrug-resistant urinary tract infections, advanced age is one of these factors (64.7% of studies) [71].

In the United States, a multicentre study carried out by Guh et al between 2012 and 2013 showed that the average age of patients with carbapenem-resistant Enterobacteriaceae infections (70% of which were urinary tract infections) was 66 years, and the age group most affected was between 65 and 79 years (31%) [26].

In our series, the average age of the patients was 57.3 years, and 43.4% of them were aged between 56 and 65 years, which is consistent with the data in the literature.

However, some studies have found no link between age and the occurrence of such infections. This is the case of a retrospective case-control study by Shilo et al, who found no significant difference in the incidence of carbapenem-resistant uropathogenic infections between elderly subjects and those under 65 years of age [72]. Lee et al. do not consider age to be a determining factor in the antibiotic resistance of enterobacteria isolated in urinary tract infections [73].

2. Gender

The incidence of urinary tract infections is higher in women than in men due to a number of anatomical and physiological factors [74].

However, according to the meta-analysis by Tenney et al, male sex is a risk factor for multi-resistant urinary tract infections (61.5%) [71]. Studies conducted in India and Germany have concluded that male sex favours infections with carbapenem-resistant pathogens *(p=0.050* and *p=0.0025* respectively) [75] [76]. Other analytical studies aimed at determining the factors favouring the occurrence of urinary tract infections, particularly those with carbapenem-resistant germs, found no difference in incidence between the sexes [72].

In an American multicentre study, 59% of patients with carbapenem-resistant Enterobacteriaceae infections (70% of which were urinary tract infections) were female [26].

Our results concur with those of the latter study. There was a predominance of women, with a sex ratio (M/F) of 0.77.

3. Comorbidities

Certain comorbidities represent a risk factor for the acquisition of urinary tract infections caused by carbapenem-resistant uropathogens, such as diabetes [26] [77], haemodialysis [78] and neoplasia [77]. This can be explained by the fact that:

- the pathology itself is a cause of alteration and weakening of the host's defence mechanisms

- the underlying pathology is the cause of frequent visits to health facilities and possible hospitalisation

- the pathology predisposes to infections, which increases the frequency of antibiotic use, particularly broad-spectrum antibiotics, which can have a significant impact on the microbiota.

Our results are consistent with the literature. In our series, the main comorbidities present in our patients were diabetes and arterial hypertension, observed in 56.5% and 39.1% respectively. Among our 23 patients, 5 (21.7%) had chronic renal failure, 2 had COPD and 2 were receiving long-term corticosteroid therapy.

3.1. Diabetes

Diabetics are at increased risk of infection. The urinary tract is the main site of infection in diabetics [79]. Several factors may contribute to the occurrence of such infections [80]:

- the high level of glucose in the urine and in the renal parenchyma, which provides a favourable environment for the development and adhesion of germs to the urothelium.

- bladder neuropathy, which impairs emptying.

- Weakening of the immune system.

Diabetes is considered to be one of the main comorbidities associated with carbapenem-resistant uropathogenic infections. In fact, two multicentre studies carried out in the United States [26] and Taiwan [77] found that 44.3% and 34.8% of patients respectively were diabetics. Mariappan et al concluded that diabetes is a risk factor for this type of infection *(p=0.036)* [75].

However, diabetes was only identified as a risk factor for multidrug-resistant urinary tract infections in 50% of the studies published between 19962016 [71].

3.2 Other co-morbidities

Other pathologies have been reported in the literature as incriminating factors in the acquisition of carbapenem-resistant enterobacterial infections, such as neoplasia, immunosuppressants, antihistamines 2 and haemodialysis. These risk factors were identified in a retrospective Turkish study of 720 patients with carbapenem-resistant *Klebsiella spp.* infection [78]. In our study, 5 patients

(21.7%) had chronic renal failure. One of these patients (4.3%) was undergoing haemodialysis. No history of neoplasia or immunosuppressive therapy was noted.

In contrast, Shilo et al concluded from a case-control study comparing 135 patients with carbapenem-resistant *Klebsiella pneumoniae* bacteriuria with 127 patients with carbapenem-sensitive bacteriuria that diabetes, renal failure, immunosuppression and liver cirrhosis are not risk factors for carbapenem-resistant urinary tract infections [72].

4. History of urinary tract infection

Several studies have shown that a history of urinary tract infection in the last 12 months is a risk factor for multidrug-resistant UTIs (including carbapenem-resistant Enterobacteriaceae) [71]. This association may be explained by the impact of the antibiotics prescribed and any hospitalisations during these infectious episodes. In our series, 13 patients (56.5%) had a history of urinary tract infection in the previous year, for which they had all required at least one hospitalisation.

5. Previous hospitalisation and stay in intensive care

A history of hospitalisation is one of the main risk factors for acquiring multi-resistant urinary tract infections [71].

An American multicentre study carried out between 2012 and 2013 found that 73.9% of patients with a history of hospitalisation in the last 30 days had developed a carbapenem-resistant infection [26].

Conversely, in a German study, previous hospitalisation in the last six months was not found to be a factor favouring the occurrence of carbapenem-resistant Enterobacteriaceae infections [76].

In our series, 78.3% of patients had a history of hospitalisation. The majority (69.6%) were admitted to the same hospital. A stay in a private clinic and in a regional hospital was noted in one case respectively.

The length of hospital stay is an important factor to take into account. The risk of developing carbapenem-resistant Enterobacteriaceae infections is proportional to the length of previous hospitalisation. A multicentre American study (2010-2011) found that 30.4% of patients with a previous long hospital stay ($\geq$ 25 days) were colonised by carbapenemase-secreting Enterobacteriaceae. This colonisation was only observed in 3.3% of patients with a short hospital stay [81]. This relationship may be explained by the fact that patients with a history of long-term hospitalisation have a high morbidity and require more or less invasive care and sometimes antibiotic treatment.

In our study, the average length of stay in hospital was 17 days (2-50 days).

A stay in an intensive care unit is one of the main risk factors for the acquisition of carbapenem-resistant urinary tract infections described in the literature [82]. This relationship may be explained by the diversity and multitude of care provided, the close and/or prolonged contact with potentially colonised patients and the frequency of antibiotic prescribing on these wards.

Among our patients, 13% had a history of a stay in a medical intensive care unit.

6. Invasive procedures

Urinary catheterisation in all its forms, whether recent or performed during a previous hospitalisation, favours the acquisition of multi-resistant urinary tract infections, particularly those resistant to carbapenems [71] [72] [26].

The favourable role of catheterisation in the occurrence of urinary tract infections is explained by :

- Chronic irritation of the ureteral mucosa by the urinary catheter [83].
- Biofilm production [84]
- The production of ureases by certain strains (*P. mirabilis, K. pneumoniae*) [85].

A duration of catheterisation ≥ 30 days is the main determinant of bacteriuria [86].

In our series, 15 patients (65.2%) were catheterised, 13 of whom had transient catheterisation and 3 patients had JJ catheterisation.

Univariate analysis showed an association between bladder catheterisation and carbapenem-resistant *Klebsiella pneumoniae* UTI (p=0.026).

Other invasive procedures have been mentioned in the literature as risk factors for all carbapenem-resistant pathogen infections, such as mechanical ventilation [75] [78], central venous catheterisation [82], cardiac catheterisation [72], endoscopic procedures [87] and surgical procedures [75].

7. Antibiotic consumption

Several studies have shown that previous antibiotic use is an important risk factor for the acquisition of multi-resistant urinary tract infections [71].

A case-control study by Shilo et al. revealed that the use of 1st generation cephalosporins and colistin favours urinary tract infections with carbapenem-resistant germs *(p=0.008 and p=0.036* respectively) [72].

Several studies have shown that previous use of carbapenems is implicated in the selection of carbapenem-resistant Enterobacteriaceae and is a main risk factor in the increased incidence of multi-resistant infections [75] [77] [78].

In our series, 20 cases (87.0%) had used antibiotics in the six months prior to the ERC urinary tract infection. The main families of antibiotics used were beta-lactams, followed by fluoroquinolones (87.0% and 39.1% respectively). A review of hospital records revealed that carbapenem-based antibiotics had been used in 11 cases (47.8%).

The ecological element is also a risk factor that should not be ignored or neglected. This determinant, little explored to date, is essentially represented by:
- antibiotics excreted in active form, which persist for a long time in the environment, and
- the use of antibiotics in veterinary practice [88].

8. Recent trip

Travel is the most important risk factor in the spread of carbapenem-resistant Enterobacteriaceae in different parts of the world.

A German retrospective study found that among 24 patients with an EPC infection, 5 had a history of a recent stay abroad (Turkey, Saudi Arabia, Russia or Luxembourg, Egypt) [76].

According to the French national epidemiological bulletin of 31 December 2015, a history of a stay abroad was found in 1131 patients with ERC infection, i.e. 47% of all cases reported during the period from 2004 to 2015. Of these patients, 40% had been hospitalised in a foreign establishment during the year preceding the isolation of ERC [89].

In our series, of the 23 patients, only 2 had a history of recent travel (Algeria and Saudi Arabia) with no hospital stay.

III. Clinical and paraclinical aspects of carbapenem-resistant Enterobacteriaceae urinary tract infections

1. Clinical aspects

1.1. Circumstances in which ERC urinary tract infections occur

The emergence of carbapenem resistance represents a further step towards pan-antibiotic resistance in Enterobacteriaceae. The first strains of ERC were hospital-acquired [90]. In a prospective cohort study conducted in the United States between March 2011 and December 2012, 127 cases of ERC infection were recorded, 40.2% of which were urinary. All of these infections were healthcare-associated. The majority of these (77.2%) occurred in patients hospitalised in intensive care units [91].

According to TEARS-Net, the European Antimicrobial Resistance Surveillance Network, 72.1% of carbapenemase-producing Enterobacteriaceae infections documented in France in 2017 were of hospital origin and 27.9% were of community origin.

A single-centre study carried out in Taiwan showed that 70.5% (n=55) of carbapenem-resistant uropathogenic infections (of which 34.8% were urinary tract infections) were nosocomial, whereas 29.5% were community-acquired [77].

The results of our study are in line with those reported in the literature. Indeed, 56.5% of ERC UTIs were healthcare-associated and 43.5% were community-acquired.

Given this alarming percentage of community-acquired urinary tract infections (CAUTIs) with carbapenem-resistant germs, the existence of risk factors for acquiring such germs must be taken into account in the empirical treatment of CAUTIs.

1.2. Clinical signs

■ **Signs of seriousness**

The clinical picture of ERC UTIs is more noisy than that of UTIs with susceptible germs. In a multicentre study involving 256 cases of infection with ERC, 75 of which were UTIs, L. Alexander et al showed that the severity of the clinical presentation is pronounced. Indeed, 84 patients (32.8%) presented with sepsis and an average APACHE II score of 21.9. Of these, 29.3% presented with septic shock [92].

A single-centre retrospective study by Lee et al. conducted in Taiwan (20062015), comparing the clinical aspects of multi-drug resistant urinary tract infections with those of susceptible germs, showed that disorders of consciousness were much more frequent in the multi-drug resistant urinary tract infection group than in the susceptible germs group (17.7% vs. 12.6%). This difference between the two groups was not statistically significant *(p* = 0.088). Furthermore, no difference was found between these two groups in terms of frequency of tachycardia (HR≥ 90 bpm) (82.3% versus 81.3%; *p*= 0.605) [93].

In a cohort study by Qureshi et al (2009-2012), altered consciousness dominated the clinical picture. It was present in 8 patients out of 21 (38.1%) with a carbapenem-resistant *Klebsiella pneumoniae* urinary tract infection [94].

■ **Fever**

During parenchymal urinary tract infections, fever is frequent and often high. Qureshi et al found that fever was present in the majority of ERC UTI cases (57.1%) [94].

Lee et al. showed that fever (T≥ 38.3° C) was present in more than half the cases of ERC UTI (57.8%). The frequency of a febrile state is similar to that found in the group presenting with a UTI with susceptible germs (57.7%; *p*= 0.98) [93].

However, a case-control study by Shilo et al. found fever in only 41% of patients with *K. pneumoniae* bacteriuria [72].

■ **Urinary signs**

Urinary signs such as urinary burning, dysuria and/or pollakiuria may be observed during ERC infections. However, these signs are not constant. Indeed, Qureshi et al. found dysuria in only 5 patients out of 21 (23.8%) with a carbapenem-resistant *Klebsiella pneumoniae* urinary tract infection [94].

In the study by Alexander L et al, 58.7% of patients with ERC UTI had leucocyturia on urine dipstick and 81.3% of these had pyuria on macroscopic examination of urine [92].

■ **Lower back pain**

The presence of back pain suggests an infection of the renal parenchyma. It is less common than fever. This may be due to the frequency of severe pyelonephritis accompanied by shock or impaired consciousness, and the presence of co-morbidities such as diabetes. Qureshi et al found low back pain in only one of 21 patients with ERC UTI [94].

The results of our study are consistent with those reported in the literature. Infection revealed sepsis and septic shock in 8 cases (34.8%). Altered general condition and altered consciousness were observed in 69.6% and 56.5% of cases respectively. Fever was observed in 18 cases (78.3%), while urinary signs and lumbar pain were noted in only 39.1% and 13% of cases respectively.

2. Biological aspects

2.1. Microbiological data

2.1.1. Leukocyturia

The microbiological diagnosis of an infection is based on the presence of bacteriuria greater than or equal to 10^3 CFU/ml for *E. coli* and $\geq 10^4$ CFU/ml for other enterobacteria in women, combined with significant leucocyturia ($\geq$ 10/mm).^{3}

A retrospective cohort study by Qureshi et al (2009- 2012), with the aim of studying the epidemiology of KPRC bacteriuria and its impact, found a leukocyturia rate $\geq 150/\text{mm}^3$ in 57% of these UTIs [94].

In our study, we found a similar result. Leukocyturia $\geq 150/\text{mm}3$ was observed in 60.9% of cases.

2.1.2. Prevalence of isolation of carbapenem-resistant strains in Enterobacteriaceae

Of the 7362 strains of Enterobacteriaceae isolated from urine during the period of our study, 34 were resistant to carbapenems, corresponding to a prevalence of 0.46%.

This result is not similar to that found in a prospective study carried out at CHU Ibn Sina Rabat, where 88 out of 3884 strains of Enterobacteriaceae isolated from urinary samples taken in the various departments of the hospital during the period from July 2012 to July 2013 were resistant to carbapenems (i.e. a prevalence of 3.64%) [95].

A multicentre cohort study (2009-2013) found that the prevalence of carbapenem-resistant strains among enterobacteria responsible for urinary tract infections in the United States was 2.9% [96].

According to the European Antibacterial Resistance Surveillance Centre

(EARS-Net), resistance to carbapenems in enterobacteria is high in some southern European countries, where it exceeds 30%, such as Greece, where the resistance rate was 67.1% in 2016. However, the spread of EPCs in France is still limited. Less than 1% of *K. pneumoniae* strains isolated in invasive infections in 2016 were resistant to carbapenems.

2.1.3. Distribution of ERC strains by germ type

In our study, *Klebsiella pneumoniae* was the most isolated germ (69.5%), followed by *Enterobacter cloacae* (26%). These results are consistent with those of numerous studies.

In a multicentre retrospective study, encompassing 22 centres in four countries (USA, UK, Italy, Greece) and conducted over a 6-month period (September 2013- March 2014), Alexander et al. found that the most frequently isolated strains in ERC UTIs were: *Klebsiella pneumoniae* in 78.7% of cases (59/75), *Enterobacter cloacae* and *Escherichia coli* in 5.3% of cases (4/75) respectively [92].

A single-centre retrospective study conducted in Taiwan (Jan 2015- June 2015) showed that the most frequently isolated ERCs during infections (a third of which were urinary tract infections) were: *K.pneumoniae* (53.8%) followed by *E. cloacae* (30.8%) [77]. However, a meta-analysis by Xu et al. of studies carried out between 2000 and 2012 to determine the epidemiological aspects of ERC infections in Asian countries showed that *K. pneumoniae* and *E. coli* were the predominant strains (39.3% and 22% respectively) [97].

A prospective cohort study conducted in the United States from March 2011 to December 2012 showed that *K. pneumoniae* was isolated in 89% of ERC infections (40.2% of which were urinary tract infections) [91].

In a study carried out as part of the microbiological and epidemiological surveillance of EPCs in Belgium (January 2012-June 2014), Jans et al showed that *K. pneumoniae, E.cloacae* and *E.coli* accounted for 65.7%, 8.3% and 8.1% of ERCs respectively (Figure 20).

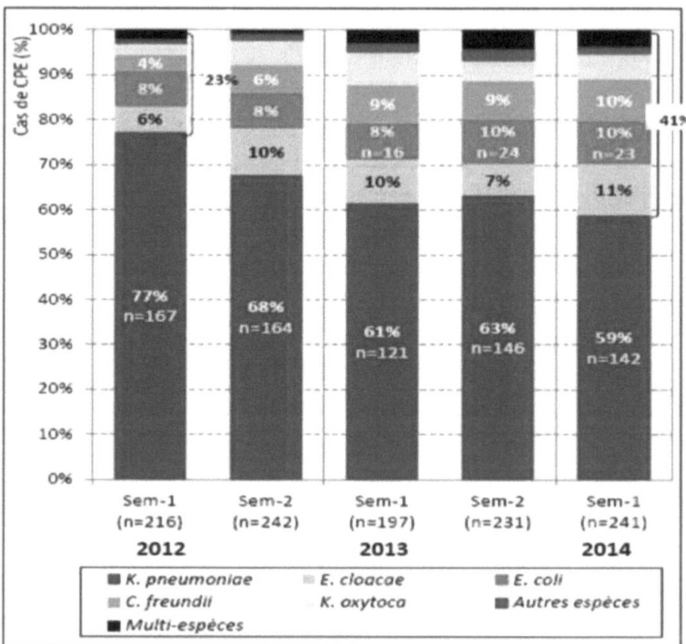

Figure 27: Distribution of EPCs by species (2012-2014) in Belgium [98].

More recently, the ERC strains isolated in France were *K. pneumoniae* in 34.2% of cases and *E.coli* in 33.9% of cases (according to EARS.Net).

2.1.4. Breakdown of strains by age and sex

In our study, there was a slight female predominance (56.5%) of *K. pneumoniae* urinary tract infections. This pathogen was isolated in half the cases from patients aged between 56 and 65 years. *E. cloacae* was isolated equally from both sexes, with no predominance of one age group.

In contrast to our results, a prospective multicentre study carried out in the USA between December 2011 and October 2013 found that the mean age of patients with carbapenem-resistant *K.pneumoniae* UTIs was 72 years and 59% of them were women [98] [99].

Shilo et al. showed that patients with carbapenem-resistant uropathogenic bacteriuria (colonisation or urinary tract infection) were on average 77 years old and 54% were female [72].

2.1.5. Strain distribution by year of isolation

In our study, 43.5% of ERC strains were isolated in 2015. *K. pneumoniae* was the most frequently isolated germ throughout the study period.

In France, there was a peak in the isolation of *K. pneumoniae* and *E. cloacae* in 2014, followed by a downward trend. The number of documented cases was the same in 2016-2017. In contrast, the trend in the frequency of isolation of other enterobacteria (*E. aerogenes, E. coli, etc.*) seems to be following an increasing curve, with a peak in 2017 [100] (Figure 21).

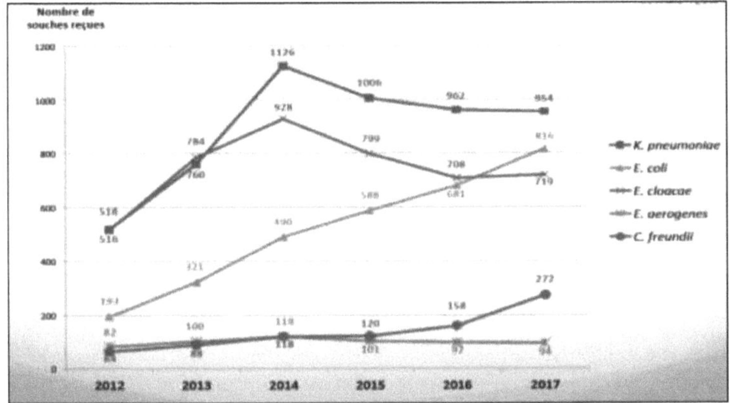

Figure 28: Trend in the number of EPC strains sent to the CNR from 2012 to 2017 [100]

2.1.6. Distribution of strains by month of isolation

In our study, 65.2% of ERC strains were isolated during the winter-spring period.

Contrary to our results, the peak incidence of ERC infections in France and Belgium was observed during the autumn (Figures 22 and 23) [98] [100].

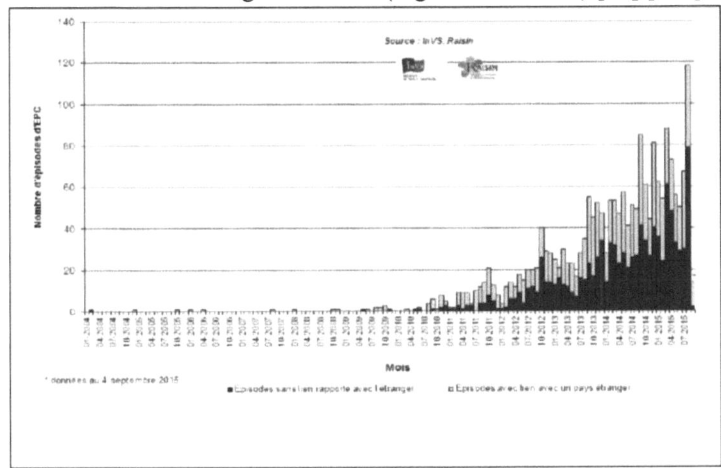

Figure 29: Change in the number of episodes of EPC infection reported per month in France from 2004 to 2015 [100].

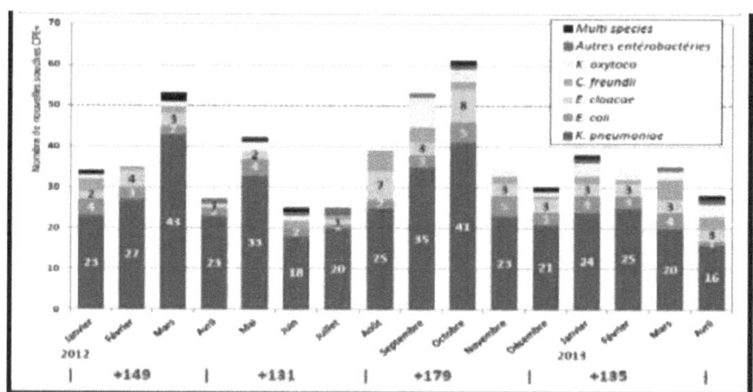

Figure 30: Monthly distribution of EPCs isolated in Belgium from 2012 to 2013[98].

2.1.7. Breakdown of strains by department

Klebsiella pneumoniae, *Enterobacter cloaceae* and *Enterobacter aerogenes*, found in our study, came mainly from intensive care units in 56.2%, 66.7% and 100% of cases respectively.

These results are consistent with those of several studies. This is the case of Carrilho's study, which showed that 77.2% of ERC strains (40.2% of which were isolated in urine) were isolated from patients hospitalised in intensive care units [91].

In a retrospective study determining the epidemiological profile of ERCs in the microbiology laboratory of Rabat University Hospital, it was found that the majority of ERCs isolated were from paediatric intensive care units and general intensive care units in 46.4% and 12.7% of cases respectively [95].

Patients hospitalised in intensive care units are at greater risk of colonisation and infection by multi-resistant pathogens, including ERCs, due to the severity of their illness, long hospital stays, frequent invasive procedures and the use of broad-spectrum antibiotics.

2.1.8. Susceptibility profile of strains to antibiotics

All carbapenem-resistant uropathogenic strains isolated in our study were resistant to all beta-lactams and fluoroquinolones. However, they were sensitive to colistin in all cases, fosfomycin and tamikacin in 20 cases (87%) respectively, tigecycline in 13 cases (56.5%), sulfonamide/trimethoprim in 4 cases (17.4%) and gentamicin in 3 cases (13%) (Table XI).

A prospective multicentre study carried out in the United States, evaluating the various therapeutic alternatives for KPRC urinary tract infections and their impact, showed a sensitivity profile for these uropathogens similar to that found in our study, with sensitivity rates of 91%, 83%, 53%, 38% and 33% respectively for colistin, tamikacin, tigecycline, gentamicin and cotrimoxazole [99].

58

In a study carried out at the microbiology department of Catania University Hospital (Italy) in 2014, Mezzatesta et al showed that carbapenemase-producing strains of *Klebsiella. Pneumoniae* strains producing carbapenemases, isolated from urinary samples, were resistant to beta-lactams and fluoroquinolones, but sensitive to fosfomycin and cotrimoxazole in 82% and 32% of cases respectively. Their sensitivity rate to nitrofurans was 28%. Contrary to the data in this study, all the ERC strains isolated in our study were resistant to nitrofurans [101].

2.1.9. Blood cultures

In our study, blood cultures were taken in 9 cases (39.1%). They were positive in 7/17 samples, four of which isolated the same bacteria with the same sensitivity profile as that isolated in the ECBU.

Van Duin et al showed that 10 patients out of 53 (18.9%) with a KPC urinary tract infection had bacteremia with the same germ [99].

In another retrospective monocentric study, Bryan, Alexander et al showed that 14% of patients had a positive blood culture for the same germ as that isolated at the ECBU, with the same sensitivity profile [102].

2.2. Other biological parameters: CBC, CRP, blood creatinine....

Lee et al, in a retrospective study covering the period from 2006 to 2015, comparing the clinical and paraclinical aspects of multidrug-resistant urinary tract infections with those of   susceptible germs ,   found that

There was   no   biological   difference   between   these   two   groups. Hyperleukocytosis ($> 12,000/mm^3$), thrombocytopenia (platelet count $<$ $100,000/mm^3$) and positive CRP (>10 mg/dl) were found in: 55.5% vs 55.9% with *p=0.918*, 13.2% vs 13.5% with *p=* 0.940 and 55% vs 54.1% with *p=* 0.853 respectively [93].

Impairment of renal function was much more frequent in the multidrug-resistant urinary tract infection group (24.5% vs 16.4%; *p=0.016*) [93].

The results of our study are similar to those found in the aforementioned study. WBC >10,000/mm3 and CRP >50 mg/dl were present in 82.6% and 69.6% of cases respectively. However, a platelet count of less than 100,000/mm3 was found in 8.7% of cases. Almost half of our patients (45.4%) had renal failure.

3. Radiological aspects

In our study, additional radiology (ultrasound and/or scenography) was performed in 78.3% of cases. The most common abnormalities were nephromegaly (hydronephrosis), dilatation of the pyelocecal cavities and urinary lithiasis in 22.7% (5/18), 22.2% (4/18) and 16.6% (3/18) of cases respectively.

These results are in line with those reported in the literature. Indeed, Lee et al showed that radiological abnormalities such as hydronephrosis, renal or ureteral iithiasis were significantly more frequent during urinary tract infections with multi-resistant germs than those with sensitive germs. These abnormalities were observed in 25% vs 15.6% ($p= 0.005$), 23.3% vs 14.3% ($p= 0.006$) and 16.4% vs 9.3% ($p= 0.011$) of cases respectively [93].

IV. Therapeutic aspects

ERC infections pose a major therapeutic problem due to the limited choice of active antibiotics and the absence of a clear consensus on the therapeutic approach.

In practice, treatment options are often limited to aminoglycosides, tigecycline, colistin, fosfomycin and even certain quinolones.

A cross-sectional study using a questionnaire distributed over the internet, aimed mainly at infectious diseases specialists in various countries around the world and covering a period of 6 months (January-June 2017), shows that almost half (48.6%) of specialists do not follow a clear and conventional therapeutic approach in the treatment of CTA infections. Indeed, the site of infection, its severity and the MIC of the antibiotic are the main factors they take into consideration when choosing antibiotic therapy [103].

1. Molecules used

In our study, the main drugs prescribed for the treatment of urinary tract infections caused by carbapenem-resistant organisms were: tamikacin, tigecycline, colistin, imipenem, fosfomycin and tazocillin (68.2%, 50.0%, 45.5%, 27.2% and 22.7% respectively).

❖ **Aminosides :**

Aminoglycosides are rapidly bactericidal antibiotics with concentration-dependent activity. They are used in severe infections or infections caused by resistant bacteria, such as ERC infections. A prospective American cohort study describing the therapeutic aspects of urinary tract infections with KPC-producing Enterobacteriaceae and their clinico-biological impact demonstrated the clinical and biological efficacy of aminoglycosides administered to seven patients (100%) [102].

Another prospective Brazilian study describing the clinical, microbiological, therapeutic and evolutionary aspects of CRT infections and their prognostic factors, involving 127 patients (40.2% of whom had a CRT urinary tract infection), showed that the use of aminoglycosides was associated with 70.4% of deaths ($p= 0.2$) [91].

In our study, gentamicin was not used due to a high rate of resistance to this antibiotic in the Enterobacteriaceae isolated. Amikacin was used in 13 cases (56.5%). It was prescribed in combination with other antibiotics in all cases. Amikacin was associated with a clinical success rate in 76.9% of cases. The difference between this rate and that of combinations not including amikacin was not statistically significant (*p=0.276*).

This result is consistent with data in the literature. In fact, in a meta-analysis by C. Lee et al, involving 30 patients with ERC infection divided into two groups: patients treated with an aminoglycoside as monotherapy (20%) vs. patients treated with an aminoglycoside in combination with other antibiotics (80%), there was no difference between the two groups in terms of clinical failure (0% vs. 17%, $p = 0.6$) [104].

❖ **Tigecycline :**

Tigecycline is a glycylcycline that is active against almost all gram-positive cocci, enterobacteria and certain anaerobic bacteria. It retains in vitro activity against a large number of multi-resistant BGN [105]. However, ERCs are showing increasing resistance to this glycylcycline. In a prospective multicentre study carried out in the United States, Van Duin et al showed that the rate of resistance of ERCs to tigecycline was 18% [106]. In another retrospective study carried out in 5 South Korean hospitals, this rate reached 14.5% [107].

It has been reported in the literature that ERC urinary tract infections treated with tigecycline are at risk of clinical failure and excess mortality. In fact, in a prospective multicentre study conducted in the United States between December 2011 and October 2013, evaluating the efficacy of antibiotics in the treatment of KPRC urinary tract infections, patients who received tigecycline had a higher risk of clinical failure *(p = 0.0425)* [99].

Furthermore, in a prospective Brazilian study of 127 patients (40.2% of whom had a urinary tract infection with ERC), the use of tigecycline was associated with 59% of deaths. However, the difference with other antibiotics was not significant *(p = 0.27)* [91].

However, other studies attest to the efficacy of high-dose tigecycline even as monotherapy in the treatment of BRC urinary tract infections; such as the case reported by K. Brust in 2014 of a patient with a history of chronic renal failure who presented with a KPRC urinary tract infection treated with high-dose tigecycline (100 mg*2/d) and who progressed well both clinically and biologically, thus confirming the success of this therapeutic option [108].

This latter therapeutic alternative appears to be frequently used; in fact, a questionnaire sent out to infectious diseases specialists worldwide revealed that high-dose tigecycline was used in almost half the cases of these infections (54.5%) [103].

The meta-analysis by C. Lee et al. showed no significant difference, in terms of therapeutic failure, between patients with ERC infections treated with tigecycline monotherapy and those treated with a combination containing this compound (29% vs. 37%; *p*= 0.4) [104].

As a result, the use of this antibiotic should be limited to situations where there are no therapeutic alternatives.

The results of our study are consistent with certain data in the literature. In fact, 11 patients had received tigecycline (as monotherapy in one case and in combination in the other cases). Four of the ten patients who had received tigecycline in combination with other antibiotics had a favourable outcome. On the other hand, the patient who received tigecycline monotherapy had an unfavourable outcome. Prescription of this antibiotic was associated with a poor prognosis (*p=0.032*).

❖ **Polymyxins :**

Polymyxins are antibiotics from the polypeptide family. They are bactericidal and active against many Gram-negative bacilli, and are considered to be among the most active agents against ERCs [109].

They are essentially represented by polymyxin E (colistin) and polymyxin B. Colistin is administered parenterally in the form of an inactive prodrug: colistimethate sodium (CMS). Only a small fraction of CMS is slowly converted into the active form of colistin, as the majority (70%) of this prodrug is eliminated by the kidneys even before it is converted into colistin [110].

Therefore, because of this slow transformation of CMS, the usefulness of a loading dose seems necessary. In fact, therapeutic concentrations are generally reached after 48 h without a loading dose and in 12 to 24 h with a loading dose [110]. Excretion of SMC depends on renal function. A patient with impaired renal function will eliminate less CMS and the fraction of the dose converted into colistin will be higher. Colistin dosage is therefore adapted to renal function. In contrast, polymyxin B administered parenterally in its active form does not require dose adjustment in cases of moderate renal impairment[111]. This galenic form is not available in many countries, including France.

In addition, high doses of colistin are essential to maximise the therapeutic effect and reduce the rate of clinical failure. Indeed, in a Greek retrospective study of 259 patients infected with ERC, the mortality rate was 21.7% for patients treated with high doses of colistin (9MUI/d) versus 27.8% and 38.6% for those treated with low doses of 3 and 6 MUI/d, respectively [112].

In the same study, therapeutic failure was noted in 90% of patients who received colistin monotherapy compared with 54.8% of those who received colistin in combination with other antibiotics (*p=0.002*) [112].

A study including 18 patients infected with KPC-producing *K. pneumoniae* showed a success rate of 66.7% for colistin alone or in combination with an aminoglycoside or tigecycline [113]. Another study found an attributable mortality of 25% with MBL strains resistant to colistin [114].

In our study, 10 patients had received colistin in combination with another antibiotic. Of these, 7 patients (70%) had a favourable outcome. This clinical success rate was not significantly different from that observed in patients who had received other antibiotic therapy ($p= 0.616$).

❖ **Fosfomycin :**

Fosfomycin is a broad-spectrum antibiotic. Its antibacterial activity includes Gram-positive cocci and BGN, including certain ESBLs and *P aeruginosa*. Carbapenem-resistant uropathogens remain sensitive to this compound.

Indeed, IV fosfomycin has been used successfully to treat multi-resistant *K. pneumoniae* infections [113].

Two studies, one prospective conducted in India over a 6-month period from November 2015 to April 2016 [115] and the other in Italy carried out at the Catania microbiology department in 2014 [101], found a sensitivity rate of 89.1% and 82% respectively for ERCs to fosfomycin.

However, this compound must be combined with one or more antibiotics, because of the increased risk of selection of resistant mutants.

A prospective Greek study demonstrated the efficacy of intravenous fosfomycin, prescribed in combination with other antibiotics, in the treatment of 11 cases of KPRC infections (including 4 urinary tract infections) [116].

In our study, fosfomycin was used as monotherapy and in combination in 2 and 3 cases respectively. This antibiotic therapy was associated with a favourable outcome in one case out of 2 when prescribed as monotherapy, and in all cases when prescribed in combination. In sum, the use of fosfomycin was effective in 80% of cases. This association with clinical success was not statistically significant *(p = 0.477)*.

❖ **Carbapenems :**

Carbapenem MICs for carbapenemase-producing strains are quite variable from one carbapenem molecule to another (tableXXVII). This variability in resistance levels has suggested the possible use of certain carbapenems in the treatment of these infections. However, higher levels of resistance to these antibiotics, acquired under treatment, have been reported [113].

Some EPC strains remain sensitive to carbapenems when the MIC does not exceed 4 to 8 mg/l [117].

Table XXVII: Susceptibility/resistance criteria for carbapenems according to American (CLSI) and European (EUCAST) recommendations [5].

	CLSI		EUCAST	
	S(≤)	R (≥)	S(≤)	R (≥)
Imipenem	4	8	2	8

Meropenem	4	8	2	8
Ertapneme	2	4	0,5	1
Doripenem	N/A	N/A	1	4

Not determined

High doses of carbapenems in continuous infusion appear to increase the bactericidal effect on ERCs [118].

In a meta-analysis, Tzouvelekis et al. showed that the mortality rate in EPC infections was lowest (8.3%) when combinations of antibiotics including at least one carbapenem were used, compared with other treatment options [119].

In addition, the combination of two carbapenems (meropenem/doripenem and ertapenem) appears to be highly effective against ERC infections. In fact, because of its affinity for carbapenemases, ertapenem inhibits these enzymes and allows the second carbapenem to act: in this combination, ertapenem acts as a "suicide substrate" [120].

A literature review by de OlaMashini et al. encompassing articles published from 1966 to March 2018, evaluating the efficacy and safety of dual carbapenem therapy in patients infected with carbapenemase-producing *Klebsiella pneumoniae* (by administration of ertapenem followed by a slow infusion of doripenem or meropenem), found that the clinical and microbiological success rate of this treatment option reached 70% of cases [121].

In our study, the combination of imipenem, ertapenem and amikacin was used in a single case with a good clinical and biological outcome.

❖**Cotrimoxazole**

Cotrimoxazole is a combination of bacteriostatic antibiotics: sulphamethoxazole and trimethoprim, which are active against gram-negative germs, including enterobacteria and gram-positive cocci.

Evaluation of the efficacy of cotrimoxazole in the treatment of KPC infections is poorly described in the literature. An Italian single-centre study, conducted between November 2012 and June 2015, showed that 9 out of 10 patients with KPC-producing *Klebsiella pneumoniae* infection treated with cotrimoxazole monotherapy had progressed well [122].

In our study, only one patient had received cotrimoxazole combined with amikacin, with a good outcome.

❖**Quinolones**

In an Australian study, the majority of enterobacterial strains producing IMP-4 remained susceptible to quinolones and four patients were successfully treated with these antibiotics [113].

2. Monotherapy or combination of antibiotics

The use of a combination of antibiotics was reported by 99.1% of infectious disease specialists questioned about their treatment options for the management of ERC infections [103].

A systematic review of the literature by Lee at al. covering articles published between 2001 and 2011 and studying the therapeutic aspects of infections with KPC-producing bacteria (10% of which were urinary tract infections) shows that clinical failure is much higher in cases treated with monotherapy than in those treated with a combination of antibiotics (49% vs 25%, $p=0.01$) [104].

In a review of 20 studies, Tzouvelekis et al showed that the mortality rate for ERC urinary tract infections was much lower when a combination of antibiotics was prescribed than when a single agent was used (27.4% vs 38.7% with $p<0.001$) [119].

However, a prospective Brazilian study describing the clinical, microbiological, therapeutic and evolutionary aspects of ERC infections (of which 40.2% were urinary tract infections), showed that the mortality rate in ERC urinary tract infections was similar to that found in the group treated with a combination of antibiotics [21% (6/28) vs 26% (6/23); $p = 0.47$] [91].

Our results are consistent with those of the latter study. Indeed, 19 patients had received a combination of antibiotics (86.4%). The clinico-biological outcome was favourable in 13 of these patients (68.4%). The most frequently prescribed combinations were: colistin-tigecycline and tigecycline-amikacin in 5 cases each, with a favourable outcome in 2 cases each (40%).

Two-thirds of our patients (66.7%) who received a single antibiotic had a good outcome. Analysis of these data shows that the prescription of a single antibiotic or a combination of antibiotics is not statistically associated with an unfavourable outcome ($p=0.705$).

Following a meta-analysis, Falagas et al. showed that the mortality rate of carbapenemase-producing *Klebsiella spp* infections (which were mainly urinary tract infections) treated with a combination of tigecycline and colistin varied from 0 to 30% [123].

In a multicentre Taiwanese study, Chang et al found that the colistin-tigecycline and tigecycline-amikacin combinations were associated with a high mortality rate (40% and 50% respectively) [124].

In addition to this fairly high mortality rate, the combination of such antibiotics increases the risk of *clostridium difficile* colonisation/infection and of adverse effects, particularly nephrotoxicity.

3. New therapeutic alternatives

The prospects for new molecules in the treatment of carbapenemase-producing

Enterobacteriaceae infections are fairly limited.

New antibiotics have shown good efficacy in the treatment of ERC infections, such as :

❖ **Ceftazidime/avibactam**

This involves combining a new beta-lactamase inhibitor (avibactam) with a 3rd generation cephalosporin (ceftazidime). Avibactam inhibits Ambler's class A and class C beta-lactamases and some class D enzymes [125]. This combination was validated by The Food and Drug Administration in February 2015 [126]. The initial data on the clinical efficacy of ceftazidime-avibactam in the treatment of urinary tract infections with ERCs come mainly from the prospective study by Vazquez et al, which compared treatment with ceftazidime/avibactam vs imipenem/cilastine in 135 patients with urinary tract infections and found no difference in efficacy between these 2 groups [127].

This combination of antibiotics is currently in phase 3 of a therapeutic trial for urinary tract and intra-abdominal ERC infections.

❖ **Meropenem-vaborbactam**

Varborbactam is the first ß-lactamase inhibitor to restore the activity of meropenem against EPCs [128].

❖ **Eravacycline**

It is a synthetic fluorocycline active against : *Escherichia coli, Klebsiella pneumoniae, Citrobacter freundii, Enterobacter cloacae, Klebsiella oxytoca, Enterococcus faecalis, Enterococcus faecium, Staphylococcus aureus, Streptococcus anginosus group, Clostridium perfringens, Bacteroides* species, *and Parabacteroides distasonis* [124]. It is indicated for complicated intra-abdominal infections. In vitro studies show that teravacycline is 2 to 4 times more active than tigecycline on ERCs [129].

Its main adverse effects are digestive, such as nausea and vomiting [124].

❖ **Plazomicin**

This is a new generation of aminoglycosides, the neoglicosides, derived from sisomicin. Its structure is similar to that of the old aminoglycosides (gentamicin, amikacin, tobramycin) but is modified by ERC enzymes [130].Approved in June 2018 by the FDA for the treatment of severe bacterial infections caused by carbapenem-resistant *Escherichia coli, Klebsiella pneumoniae, Proteus mirabilis, Enterobacter cloacae*, particularly in complicated urinary tract infections (pyelonephritis), in adult patients for whom other options are reduced or impossible.

The efficacy of plazomicin on ERCs has been shown to be superior to that of the older aminoglycosides [131].

Its main adverse effects are neurological and renal [124].

V. Impact of IU at ERC

1. Length of hospital stay

The average length of hospital stay after the onset of infection was 25.5 days (4-100 days) in our study. This is far longer than that found in other studies. In fact, in a multicentre retrospective study conducted in 4 countries (the United States, the United Kingdom, Greece and Italy) between September 2013 and March 2014, the average length of hospitalisation for urinary tract infections with ERCs was 8.2 +/- 12.7 days [92]. This was 18 days (8- 28.5 days) in a Brazilian prospective study of 127 patients with CRF infection (40.2% of which were urinary tract infections) [91].

It can be deduced that urinary tract infections associated with CRTs are associated with long hospital stays due to the frequency of complications that may arise during their course.

2. Morbidity/mortality

In a meta-analysis by Xu et al of articles published up to December 2015 estimating mortality in patients with carbapenem-resistant *Klebsiella pneumoniae* infections, the mortality rate for KPRC urinary tract infections was 13.5% compared with 54.3% for KPRC bacteraemia. In this meta-analysis, the overall mortality rate for KPRC infections was 33.2%, 46.7%, 50.1% and 44.8% respectively in North America, South America, Europe and Asia [132].

Alexander et al found in a multicentre study that the 28-day mortality rate for ERC urinary tract infections was 17.3% [92].

Death was noted in 27.3% of ERC urinary tract infections compared with 61.4% of ERC pneumonia in a prospective Brazilian study (2011-2012) [91].

These results are similar to those found in our series, where the death rate was 30.4% (13.0% was related to the infection).

Factors predictive of poor prognosis identified in the literature include :

- advanced age :

In a prospective Brazilian study of 127 patients with ERC infection (40.2% of whom were urinary tract infections), advanced age ($\geq$ 60 years) was associated with 56.8% of deaths *(p = 0.06)* [91]. In our study, advanced age was not a factor in poor prognosis *(p = 0.253)*.

- The presence of co-morbidities :

In our series, the presence of a comorbidity (diabetes, renal failure or other) was not associated with a poor prognosis *(p > 0.05)*. This result is not consistent with the literature. In a multicentre study, Alexander et al showed that chronic renal failure and haemodialysis were associated with a mortality rate of 33.3% and 41.2% respectively on day 28 of 256 cases of ERC infection (75 of which were urinary) [92].

Carrilho et al. found in a prospective study that haemodialysis alone constituted a risk factor for mortality during CRF infections (40.2% of which were urinary) of *(p=0.04)* [91].

In a multicentre Taiwanese study, diabetes was also found to be a poor prognostic factor in ERC infections (*p* = 0.04) (10.6% of which were urinary) [124].

- <u>Admission to the intensive care unit :</u>

In a meta-analysis by Xu et al., admission to an intensive care unit for KPRC infections was associated with a high mortality rate (48.9%) [132]. In our study, admission to the intensive care unit was associated with an unfavourable outcome in 50% of cases (*p* = 0.069).

- <u>Severe sepsis or septic shock:</u>

In the study by Alexander et al, mortality on the 28th day following severe sepsis and secondary septic shock in 256 cases of ERC infections (including 75 urinary tract infections) was 44% and 46.7% respectively [92].

The study by Carrilho et al concluded that septic shock was a predictive factor for mortality *(p* = 0.0002) [91].

The same is true of the Taiwanese multicentre study by Chang et al, which, following a multivariate analysis, showed an association between septic shock and 30-day mortality in ERC infections (*p=0.04*) [124].

In our series, the presence of severe sepsis or septic shock was associated with a poor prognosis *(p* = 0.026).

- <u>Inappropriate empirical antibiotic therapy :</u>

In a multicentre American study (2009-2013), inappropriate empirical antibiotic therapy prescribed for ERC and ESC infections was associated with a mortality rate of 52.8% and 11.1% respectively [96].

In our series, inappropriate empirical antibiotic therapy was noted in 8 cases. Of these, 3 cases (37.5%) had an unfavourable outcome. Statistical analysis found no relationship between empirical antibiotic therapy and prognosis (*p=0.510*).

- <u>Time between onset of clinical signs and effective antibiotic therapy > 2 days:</u>

In a study by Chang et al, active antibiotic therapy initiated within the first 48 hours of ERC infection was associated with a 30-day survival rate of 91.3% [124]. In our series, this rate was 75%. Statistical analysis showed no association between this delay and the mortality rate (*p*= 0.963).

3. Cost

ERC UTIs have economic consequences, both in terms of the complications they can cause clinically and the measures put in place to limit their spread.

In fact, in a multicentre retrospective American study (2009-2013), the average overall cost of managing urinary tract infections caused by ERC versus those caused by ESC was \$33,400 and \$19,036 respectively (p<0.001) [96].

These results are not consistent with those found in our study. In fact, the average overall cost of managing UTIs in ERC was 3875.5 DT (1356.4 dollars).

- I. Prevention

The growing incidence of ERC infections, raising fears of therapeutic impasses, is prompting us to rigorously apply prevention and control measures to limit their emergence and prevent epidemic outbreaks.

Controlling the spread of ERCs is based on a dual strategy of :

- reducing the prescription of antibiotics in order to limit selection pressure and

- prevention of spread from carrier patients.

In fact, preventive measures according to international guidelines [133] [134] [135] are essentially based on 4 aspects:

- Rational use of antibiotics
- Reporting infected or colonised cases
- Identification of ERC carriers (screening)
- Hygiene measures, particularly hand hygiene.

1. Rational use of antibiotics

Inappropriate use of antibiotics encourages the emergence of multi-resistant microorganisms such as ERC. Proper use of antibiotics can reduce the incidence of infections caused by these bacteria. It is based on : Adherence to the principles of antibiotic prescribing:

*   take into account the type of infection, the presumed causal agent, the terrain, and the pharmacokinetics and pharmacodynamics of the compound used.

*   use doses adapted to each situation and adjusted according to the condition of the patient (sepsis, renal failure, etc.)

*   avoid unnecessary prolongation of antibiotic therapy

*adapt antibiotic therapy to the antibiogram data

*   evaluate antibiotic therapy after 48 to 72 hours.

2. Reporting infected or colonised cases

Any case of urinary tract infection or colonisation with ERC must be reported in order to - take the necessary preventive measures

-be able to assess the epidemiological situation in the department, within the establishment and at national level.

The alert must be mentioned in each volume of the medical record and in the computerised admission system, if available.

In our study, reporting of ERC cases was not automated. In fact, mention of the presence of an ERC infection was limited to medical records and surveillance forms.

3. Identification of ERC carriers (Screening)

Screening patients who are carriers of such micro-organisms (such as urinary ERC colonisation) is strongly recommended:

J On admission :

-patients hospitalised for 24 hours or more in an endemic country in the last year, or in a healthcare establishment that has had an outbreak of CRA in the last 3 months

-patients who have had close contact with carrier patients

-patients known to be carriers

J During hospitalisation :

-patients who have had contact with a carrier.

-patients hospitalised in a care unit where ERCs have been reported or where there is a significant epidemiological risk.

Healthy carriers are detected by rectal swab analysis or stool analysis in at-risk patients. Chromagar KPC medium (Chromagar, France) allows good detection of strains expressing KPC. ChromID ESBLs medium contains a selective cephalosporin. It allows the detection of any strain with a certain degree of cephalosporin resistance. Insofar as most strains with a carbapenemase are also resistant to cephalosporins, this medium is currently the most suitable for detecting carriers of strains producing a carbapenemase. Only *K. pneumoniae* strains expressing only OXA-48 without associated ESBL would not be isolated on this selective medium. The time taken to obtain results using these screening techniques is 48 hours. Some studies have indicated the value of PCR techniques for screening stools directly for carriers of KPC strains [136] [137].

4. Other measures to limit transmission

J **Patient isolation :**

Isolation must be practised for all infected or colonised patients and for patients who have had close contact with a carrier case when contact transmission precautions were not applied. Isolation must be both technical and geographical:

- Geographical isolation: isolation in a single room
- Technical isolation: wearing gowns and gloves ...

J **Hygiene :**

Good hospital hygiene practices are a cornerstone of ERC control

*Hand **hygiene**

It is the simplest and most effective preventive measure for preventing the transmission of ERCs (especially EPCs). It should be carried out by washing hands with soap and water (in the event of contact with a biological product)

and, above all, by using hydro-alcoholic friction.

* <u>Long-sleeved gowns and single-use gloves are worn on entering the room.</u>
* <u>Transport of urine samples and linen in sealed packaging</u>
* <u>Disinfection of the room after discharge.</u>

urinary tract infections (UTIs) are posing more and more therapeutic management problems due to the emergence of carbapenem-resistant enterobacteria, particularly those producing carbapenemases.

The aim of our work was to determine the epidemiological, clinical, biological, therapeutic and evolutionary characteristics of carbapenem-resistant enterobacterial urinary tract infections in our region, and to identify the factors linked to the selection of these resistant strains.

In order to meet these objectives, we conducted a retrospective study of 23 patients hospitalized in the wards of the Taher Sfar University Hospital of Mahdia, during the period from January 1, 2014 to April 30, 2018, in whom the diagnosis of ERC urinary tract infection was retained.

In this study, we included all patients with a clinical picture suggestive of a urinary tract infection and a cytobacteriological examination of the urine isolating carbapenem-resistant bacteria.

We excluded all patients with carbapenem-resistant urinary tract colonisation.

All the patients included were investigated using a pre-established data collection form, including epidemiological, clinical, paraclinical, therapeutic and evolutionary characteristics.

❖ Epidemiologically, the mean age of patients was 57.35 +/17.01 years, with extremes ranging from 18 to 80 years. A slight female predominance was noted (56.5%). Almost half the cases (43.5%) were aged between 56 and 65. One third of patients were aged over 65.

Thirteen patients (52.2%) had diabetes, 92.3% of them type 2.

Risk factors for UTI complications were present in 10 (43.5%) patients: lithiasis in 6 cases (26.1%), prostate adenoma with post-micturition residual in 2 cases, and end-stage renal disease and malformative uropathy in one case each.

Risk factors for carriage of a CRF were noted in 22 patients (95.7%). They were dominated by antibiotic therapy and hospitalisation within the last six months in 87% and 78.3% respectively. Other factors were a history of invasive procedures (65.2%), a urinary tract infection (56.5%) or surgery (26.1%) within the last 6 months, and travel in 2 cases.

❖ Clinically, fever was present in 78.3% of patients. Spontaneous and/or provoked back pain was present in 6 patients (26.1%). Nine patients (39.1%) had at least one urinary sign. Burning was the most frequent urinary sign (39.1%), followed by pollakiuria (21.7%) and dysuria (17.4%). The rectal examination was performed in only half the men. It was painless in all cases, allowing the diagnosis of prostatitis to be ruled out.

Signs of severity were present in 69.6% of cases. These were monkeys with sepsis and septic shock in 34.8% of cases respectively.

❖ Biologically, signs of severity were present in 9 cases (39.13%). These were hypoxaemia (4.3%), hyperbilirubinaemia (8.7%), acute renal failure (21.7%), haemostasis disorders (30%), metabolic acidosis (30.4%) and lacataemia ≥ 2 mmol/l (39.1%).

Bacteriologically, the uropathogens isolated were *Klebsiella pneumoniae* in 69.6% of cases, *Enterobacter cloacae* in 26.1% and *Enterobacter aerogenes* in a single case. These germs were of community origin in 10 cases (43.5%) and healthcare-associated in 13 cases (56.5%).

These ERCs were mainly isolated from patients hospitalised in intensive care.

They were all sensitive to colistin. Their resistance to amikacin and fosfomycin was 13%. Lower sensitivity was noted for tigecycline (56.5%), cotrimoxazole (17.4%) and gentamicin (13.0%). All the strains isolated were resistant to nitrofurans.

Analysis of our data showed that the only factor associated with ERC isolation was bladder catheterisation.

❖ Radiologically, renal ultrasound was performed in 18 patients (78.3%) revealing an abnormality in 6 patients. These were mainly ureteropyelocal dilatation in 5 cases (21.7%) and lithiasis in 3 cases (13%). Uroscans were performed in 3 cases and revealed ureteropylocele dilatation in all and renal lithiasis in 2 cases (8.7%). Ultrasonography of the prostate was performed in 40% of the men. It revealed prostatic hypertrophy in one case.

At the end of the clinical, biological and radiological work-up, the diagnosis was cystitis in one case, pyelonephritis in 52.2% of cases and male urinary tract infection in 43.5% of cases. The UTI was severe in 69.6% of cases. Sepsis occurred in 34.5% of cases, one of which was complicated by a secondary pulmonary site.

❖ Therapeutically, emiprical antibiotic therapy was initiated in 95.6% of cases. In fact, one patient died before initiation of antibiotic therapy. The mean time between onset of clinical signs and initiation of active antibiotic therapy was 5.6 +/- 3.2 days, with extremes ranging from 2 to 12 days. The first-line drugs prescribed were dominated by Lamikacin, tigecycline and colimycin in (68.2%), (50%) and (45.5%) of cases respectively. Adjustment of antibiotic therapy was necessary in 95.6% of cases. Therapeutic escalation was used in all cases. Monotherapy was prescribed in 13.6% of cases. The most commonly used combinations were colimycin + tigecycline and tigecycline + amikacin in 5 cases (22.7%) respectively. A combination of cotrimoxazole and Lamikacin was used in one case. Triple antibiotic therapy combining ertapenem-imipenem and amikacin was initiated in one case. The average duration of the combination was

5.2 +/- 2.2 days, with extremes ranging from 3 to 10 days.

The average duration of treatment in hospital was 25.5 days, with extremes ranging from 4 to 100 days. There was no association between bacterial species and duration of antibiotic treatment *(p=0.503)*.

❖ In terms of outcome, 15 patients had a favourable outcome (65.2%).

The mean time to disappearance of functional signs was 3 +/- 0.63 days, with extremes ranging from 2 to 4 days. Lasting apyrexia was achieved in 2.8 days, with extremes ranging from 2 to 4 days.

Death occurred in seven cases (30.4%), of which 3 (13%) were due to refractory septic shock. The mean time from onset of clinical presentation of carbapenem-resistant Enterobacteriaceae UTI to death was 41.1 +/- 36.5 days, with extremes ranging from 4 to 100 days.

No association was found between the prescription of monotherapy and an unfavourable outcome *(p=0.7)*. Prescription of tigecycline was significantly associated with an unfavourable outcome *(p=0.032)*.

❖ On the economic front :

The overall cost of managing these ERC UTIs was on average 3334.4 DT +/- 2844.9 with extremes ranging from 234.0 - 11149.2 DT.

Overall, analysis of these data shows no difference in clinical, biological, evolutionary or financial impact between *K pneumoniae* and *Enterobacter* infections.

However, our small number of patients does not allow us to draw any definitive conclusions about the epidemiological, clinical, paraclinical and evolutionary particularities of carbapenem-resistant enterobacterial urinary tract infections.

To conclude,

The rapid emergence of community strains of ERC has become a major public health problem.

Controlling the spread of these strains relies on :

* d' on the one hand, the identification of carriers through systematic research into risk factors for the carriage of carbapenemase-producing strains

* compliance with hygiene measures, in particular hand hygiene, and

* the proper use of antibiotics, particularly carbapenems.

Rationalising the use of antibiotics and epidemiological surveillance are cornerstones in the fight against the threatening increase in carbapenem resistance in enterobacteria.

1. **SPILF**.Recommendations for the management of bacterial urinary tract infections in adults. http://www.infectiologie.com/UserFiles/File/spilf/recos/infections-urinaires-spilf-argumentaire.pdf; accessed 20 August 2018.

2. **Wolff M, Joly-Guillou ML, Pajot** O. Carbapenems. Réanimation. 2009 ; 18: S199-208.

3. **Dortet L, Poirel L, Nordmann P**. Epidemiology, detection and identification of carbapenemase-producing Enterobacteriaceae. Feuill Biol. 2013; 4(312): 1-12.

4. **Gutmann L and Williamson R**. Med Sci. 1987; 3(2): 75-81.

5. **Boutet-Dubois A, Pantel A, Sotto A, Lavigne JP.** Carbapenemase-producing Enterobacteriaceae. Synthesis. https://docplayer.fr/8564683- Alin-as-les-enterobacteries-productrices-de-carbapenemases- synthese.html, accessed 25 August 2018.

6. **Bush K, JacobyGA**. Updated Functional Classification of BetaLactamases. Antimicrob Agents Chemother. 2010; 54 (3): 969-76.

7. **Ambler RP.** The Structure of beta-Lactamases. Philos Trans R Soc B-Biol Sci. 1980 ; 289 (1036): 321-31.

8. **Queenan AM, Bush K**. Carbapenemases: The Versatile β-Lactamases. Clin Microbiol Rev. 2007; 20 (3): 440-58.

9. **Yigit H, Queenan AM, Anderson GJ, Domenech-Sanchez A, BiddleJ-W, Steward C-D, Alberti S, Bush K, Tenover F-C.** Novel Carbapenem-Hydrolyzing -Lactamase, KPC-1, from a Carbapenem-Resistant Strain of *Klebsiella Pneumoniae*. Antimicrob Agents Chemother. 2001 ; 45 (4): 1151-61.

10. **Yong D, Mark AT, Christian CG, Cho HS, Sundman K, Lee K, Walsh TR**. Characterization of a New Metallo-β-Lactamase Gene, blaNDM-1, and a Novel Erythromycin Esterase Gene Carried on a Unique Genetic Structure in *Klebsiella pneumoniae* Sequence Type 14 from India. Antimicrob Agents Chemother. 2009; 53 (12): 5046-54.

11. **Perry JD, Naqvi SH, Mirza IA, Alizai SA, Hussain A, Ghirardi S et al.** Prevalence of Faecal Carriage of *Enterobacteriaceae* with NDM-1 Carbapenemase at Military Hospitals in Pakistan, and Evaluation of Two Chromogenic Media. J Antimicrob Chemother. 2011 ; 66 (10): 2288-94.

12. **Walsh TR, Weeks J, Livermore DM, Toleman MA**. Dissemination of NDM-1 Positive Bacteria in the New Delhi Environment and Its Implications for Human Health: An Environmental Point Prevalence Study - Dimensions. Lancet Infect Dis. 2011; 11(5):355-62.

13. **Poirel L, Héritier C, Tolün V, Nordmann P**. Emergence of Oxacillinase-

Mediated Resistance to Imipenem in *Klebsiella pneumoniae*. Antimicrob Agents Chemother. 2004 ; 48 (1): 15-22.

14. **Carrer A, Poirel L, Yilmaz M, Akan OA, Feriha C, Cuzon G, Matar G, Honderlick P, Nordmann P.** Spread of OXA-48-Encoding Plasmid in Turkey and Beyond. Antimicrob Agents Chemother. 2010 ; 54 (3): 136973.

15. **Neuwirth C, Siébor E, Duez JM, Péchinot A, Kazmierczak A.** Imipenem Resistance in Clinical Isolates of *Proteus Mirabilis* Associated with Alterations in Penicillin-Binding Proteins. J Antimicrob Chemother. 1995 ; 36 (2): 335-42.

16. **Yigit H, Anderson GJ, Biddle JW, Steward CD, Rasheed JK, Valera LL, McGowan JE Jr, Tenover FC.** Carbapenem resistance in a clinical isolate of *Enterobacter aerogenes* is associated with decreased expression of OmpF and OmpC porin analogs. Antimicrob Agents Chemother. 2002; 46(12):3817-22.

17. **Mainardi JL, Mugnier P, Coutrot A, Buu-Hoï A, Collatz E, Gutmann L.** Carbapenem Resistance in a Clinical Isolate of *Citrobacter Freundii*. Antimicrob Agents Chemother. 1997; 41 (11): 2352-54.

18. **Jacoby GA, Mills DM, Chow N.** Role of -Lactamases and Porins in Resistance to Ertapenem and Other -Lactams in *Klebsiella Pneumoniae*. Antimicrob Agents Chemother. 2004; 48 (8): 3203-6.

19. **Poirel L, Héritier C, Spicq C, Nordmann P.** In Vivo Acquisition of High-Level Resistance to Imipenem in *Escherichia coli*. J Clinic Microbiol. 2004 ; 42 (8): 3831-33.

20. **Armand-Lefèvre L, Leflon-Guibout V, Bredin J, Barguellil F, Amor A, Pagès JM, Nicolas-Chanoine MH.** Imipenem Resistance in *Salmonella* enterica Serovar Wien Related to Porin Loss and CMY-4 β- Lactamase Production. Antimicrob Agents Chemother. 2003; 47 (3): 1165-68.

21. **Gülmez D, Woodford N, Palepou MF, Mushtaq S, Metan G, Yakupogullari Y et al.** Carbapenem-Resistant *Escherichia Coli* and *Klebsiella Pneumoniae* Isolates from Turkey with OXA-48-like Carbapenemases and Outer Membrane Protein Loss. Int J Antimicrob Agents. 2008 ; 31 (6): 523-26.

22. **Cagnacci S1, Gualco L, Roveta S, Mannelli S, Borgianni L, Docquier JD et al.** Bloodstream Infections Caused by Multidrug-Resistant *Klebsiella Pneumoniae* Producing the Carbapenem-Hydrolysing VIM-1 Metallo- -Lactamase: First Italian Outbreak. J Antimicrob Chemother. 2007 ; 61 (2): 296-300.

23. **Landman, D, Bratu S, Quale J.** Contribution of OmpK36 to Carbapenem Susceptibility in KPC-Producing *Klebsiella Pneumoniae*. J Med Microbiol. 2009; 58 (10): 1303-8.

24. **Poirel L, Pitout JD, Nordmann P.** Carbapenemases: Molecular Diversity and Clinical Consequences. Future Microbiol. 2007; 2 (5): 501-12.

25. **Livorsi DJ, Chorazy ML, Schweizer ML, Balkenende EC, Blevins AE, Nair R et al.** A Systematic Review of the Epidemiology of Carbapenem-Resistant *Enterobacteriaceae* in the United States. Antimicrob Resist Infect Control. 2018 ; 7 :55.

26. **Guh AY, Bulens SN, Mu Y, Jacob JT, Reno J, Scott J et al.** Epidemiology of Carbapenem-Resistant *Enterobacteriaceae* in 7 US Communities, 2012-2013. JAMA. 2015 ; 314 (14): 1479-87.

27. **Bratu S, Mooty M, Nichani S, Landman D, Gullans C, Pettinato B et al.** Emergence of KPC-Possessing *Klebsiella Pneumoniae* in Brooklyn, New York: Epidemiology and Recommendations for Detection. Antimicrob Agents Chemother. 2005; 49 (7): 3018-20.

28. **Robledo IE, Vázquez GJ, Moland ES, Aquino EE, Goering RV, Thomson KS et al.** Dissemination and Molecular Epidemiology of KPC-Producing Klebsiella Pneumoniae Collected in Puerto Rico Medical Center Hospitals during a 1-Year Period. Epidemiology Research International. South Med J. 2011; 104 :40-5.

29. **Córdova E, Lespada MI, Gómez N, Pasterán F, Oviedo V, Rodríguez-Ismael C.** Clinical and epidemiological study of an outbreak of KPC- producing *Klebsiella pneumoniae* infection in Buenos Aires, Argentina. Enferm Infeccmicrobiol Clín. 2012; 30 (7): 376-79.

30. **Abboud CS, Bergamasco MD, Doi AM, Zandonadi EC, Barbosa V, Cortez D et al.** First Report of Investigation into an Outbreak Due to Carbapenemase-Producing *Klebsiella Pneumoniae* in a Tertiary Brazilian Hospital, with Extension to a Patient in the Community. J Infect Prev. 2011 ; 12 (4): 150-53.

31. **Albiger B, Glasner C, Struelens MJ, Grundmann H, Monnet DL, European Survey of Carbapenemase-Producing Enterobacteriaceae (EuSCAPE) working group.** Carbapenemase-producing *Enterobacteriaceae* in Europe: assessment by national experts from 38 countries, May 2015.Euro Surveill. 2015; 20 (45): pii=30062.

32. **Tsakris A, Kristo I, Poulou A, Markou F, Ikonomidis A, Pournaras S.** First Occurrence of KPC-2-Possessing *Klebsiella Pneumoniae* in a Greek Hospital and Recommendation for Detection with Boronic Acid Disc Tests. J Antimicrob Chemother. 2008 ; 62 (6): 1257-60.

33. **Spyropoulou A, Papadimitriou-Olivgeris M, Bartzavali C, Vamvakopoulou S, Marangos M, Spiliopoulou I et al.** A Ten-Year Surveillance Study of Carbapenemase-Producing *Klebsiella Pneumoniae* in a Tertiary Care Greek University Hospital: Predominance of KPC- over VIM- or NDM-Producing Isolates. J Med Microbiol. 2016; 65 (3): 24046.

34. **Giani T, D'Andrea MM, Pecile P, Borgianni L, Nicoletti P, Tonelli F, Bartoloni A, Rossolini GM.** Emergence in Italy of *Klebsiella Pneumoniae* Sequence Type 258 Producing KPC-3 Carbapenemase. J Clin Microbiol. 2009 ; 47 (11): 3793-94.

35. **Gaibani P, Ambretti S, Berlingeri A, Gelsomino F, Bielli A, Landini MP, Sambri V.** Rapid increase of carbapenemase-producing *Klebsiella pneumoniae* strains in a large Italian hospital. Euro Surveil. 2011 ; 16 (8). Pii : 19800.

36. **Leavitt A, Navon-Venezia S, Chmelnitsky I, Schwaber MJ, Carmeli Y.** Emergence of KPC-2 and KPC-3 in Carbapenem-Resistant *Klebsiella pneumoniae* Strains in an Israeli Hospital. Antimicrob Agents Chemother.2007; 51 (8): 3026-29.

37. **Schwaber MJ, Carmeli Y.** An Ongoing National Intervention to Contain the Spread of Carbapenem-Resistant *Enterobacteriaceae*. Clin Infect Dis. 2014; 58 (5): 697-703.

38. **Zhang Y, Wang Q, Yin Y, Chen H, Jin L, Gu B et al.** Epidemiology of Carbapenem-Resistant *enterobacteriacae* Infections: Report from the China CRE Network. Antimicrob Agents Chemother. 2008 ; 62 (2) pii: e01882-17.

39. **Qi Y, Wei Z, Ji S, Du X, Shen P, Yu Y.** ST11, the Dominant Clone of KPC-Producing *Klebsiella Pneumoniae* in China. J Antimicrob Chemother. 2011 ; 66 (2): 307-12.

40. **Kumarasamy KK1, Toleman MA, Walsh TR, Bagaria J, Butt F, Balakrishnan R et al.** Emergence of a New Antibiotic Resistance Mechanism in India, Pakistan, and the UK: A Molecular, Biological, and Epidemiological Study. Lancet Infect Dis.2010 ; 10 (9): 597-602.

41. **Seema K, Ranjan Sen M, Upadhyay S, Bhattacharjee A.** Dissemination of the New Delhi Metallo-β-Lactamase-1 (NDM-I) among *Enterobacteriaceae* in a Tertiary Referral Hospital in North India. J Antimicrob Chemother. 2011; 66 (7): 1646-47.

42. **Zhou G, Guo S, Luo Y, Ye L, Song Y, Sun G, Guo L, Chen Y, Han L, Yang J.** NDM-1 -producing Strains, Family *Enterobacteriaceae,* in Hospital, Beijing, China. Emerg Infect Dis. 2014; 20 (2): 340-42.

43. **Pisney L , Barron M, Jackson Janelle S, Bamberg W.** Notes the field: hospital outbreak of carbapenem-resistant *Klebsiella pneumoniae* producing New Delhi metallo-beta-lactamase--Denver, Colorado, 2012. MMWR Morb Mortal Wkly Rep. 2013; 62(6):108.

44. **Villegas MV, Pallares CJ, Escandón-Vargas K, Hernández-Gómez C, Correa A, Álvarez C et al.** Characterization and Clinical Impact of Bloodstream Infection Caused by Carbapenemase-Producing

Enterobacteriaceae in Seven Latin American Countries. PLoS ONE. 2016 ; 11 (4): e0154092.

45. **de Araujo CF, Silva DM, Carneiro MT, Ribeiro S, Fontana-Maurell M, Alvarez P et al.** Detection of Carbapenemase Genes in Aquatic Environments in Rio de Janeiro, Brazil. Antimicrob Agents Chemother. 2016; 60 (7): 4380-83.

46. **Zahedi Bialvaei A, Samadi Kafil H, Ebrahimzadeh Leylabadlo H, Asgharzadeh M, Aghazadeh M.** Dissemination of carbapenemases producing Gram negative bacteria in the Middle East. Iran J Microbiol. 2015 ; 7 (5): 226-46.

47. **Poirel L, Potron A, Nordmann P.** OXA-48-like carbapenemases: The phantom menace. J Antimicrob Chemother. 2012; 67(7):1597-606.

48. **Logan LK, WeinsteinRA.**The Epidemiology of Carbapenem-Resistant *Enterobacteriaceae*: The Impact and Evolution of a Global Menace. J Infect Dis. 2017; 215(suppl1):S28-S36.

49. **Manenzhe RI, Zar HJ, Nicol MP, Kaba M.** The Spread of Carbapenemase-Producing Bacteria in Africa: A Systematic Review. J Antimicrob Chemother. 2015; 70 (1): 23-40.

50. **Metwally L, Gomaa N, Attallah M, Kamel N.** High Prevalence of *Klebsiella Pneumoniae* Carbapenemase-Mediated Resistance in K. Pneumoniae Isolates from Egypt. East Mediterr Health J. 2013; 19 (11): 947-52.

51. **Mushi MF, Mshana SE, Imirzalioglu C, Bwanga F.** Carbapenemase Genes among Multidrug Resistant Gram Negative Clinical Isolates from a Tertiary Hospital in Mwanza, Tanzania. BioMed Res Int. 2014 ; 303104 :1-6.

52. **Poirel L, Revathi G, Bernabeu S, Nordmann P.** Detection of NDM-1-Producing *Klebsiella Pneumoniae* in Kenya. Antimicrob Agents Chemother. 2011 ; 55 (2): 934-36.

53. **Barguigua A, El Otmani F, Talmi M, Zerouali K, Timinouni M.** Emergence of Carbapenem-Resistant *Enterobacteriaceae* Isolates in the Moroccan Community. Diagn Micr Infec Dis. 2012 ; 73 (3): 290-91.

54. **Barguigua A, El Otmani F, Talmi M, Zerouali K, Timinouni M.** Prevalence and Types of Extended Spectrum β-Lactamases among Urinary *Escherichia Coli* Isolates in Moroccan Community. Microb Pathog.2013; 61-62: 16-22.

55. **Chouchani C1, Marrakchi R, Ferchichi L, El Salabi A, Walsh TR.** VIM and IMP Metallo-β-Lactamases and Other Extended-Spectrum β- Lactamases in *Escherichia Coli* and *Klebsiella Pneumoniae* from Environmental Samples in a Tunisian Hospital: VIM AND IMP METALLO-β-LACTAMASES. APMIS. 2011 ; 119 (10): 725-32.

56. **Leski TA, Bangura U, Jimmy DH, Ansumana R, Lizewski SE, Li RW,**

Stenger DA, Taitt CR, Vora GJ. Identification of blaOXA-51-like, blaOXA-58, blaDIM-1, and blaVIM Carbapenemase Genes in Hospital *Enterobacteriaceae* Isolates from Sierra Leone. J Clin Microbiol. 2013; 51 (7): 2435-38.

57. **Brink AJ, Coetzee J, Corcoran C, Clay CG, Hari-Makkan D, Jacobson RK et al.** Emergence of OXA-48 and OXA-181 Carbapenemases among *Enterobacteriaceae* in South Africa and Evidence of In Vivo Selection of Colistin Resistance as a Consequence of Selective Decontamination of the Gastrointestinal Tract. J Clin Microbiol. 2013; 51 (1): 369-72.

58. **Mnif B, Ktari S, Chaari A, Medhioub F, Rhimi F, Bouaziz M et al.** Nosocomial Dissemination of *Providencia Stuartii* Isolates Carrying BlaOXA-48, BlaPER-1, BlaCMY-4 and QnrA6 in a Tunisian Hospital. J Antimicrob Chemother. 2013; 68 (2): 329-32.

59. **Ktari S, Mnif B, Louati F, Rekik S, Mezghani S, Mahjoubi F et al.** Spread of *Klebsiella Pneumoniae* Isolates Producing OXA-48 -Lactamase in a Tunisian University Hospital. J Antimicrob Chemother. 2014; 66 (7): 1644-46.

60. **Mansour W, Haenni M, Saras E, Grami R, Mani Y, Ben Haj Khalifa A et al.** Outbreak of Colistin-Resistant Carbapenemase-Producing *Klebsiella Pneumoniae* in Tunisia. J Glob Antimicrob Res. 2017; 10: 8894.

61. **Ouertani R, Ben Jomàa-Jemili M, Gharsa H, Limelette A, Guillard T, Brasme L et al.** Prevalence of a New Variant OXA-204 and OXA-48 Carbapenemases Plasmids Encoded in *Klebsiella Pneumoniae* Clinical Isolates in Tunisia. Microb Drug Resist. 2018; 24 (2): 142-49.

62. **Ktari S, Arlet G, Mnif B, Gautier V, Mahjoubi F, Ben Jmeaa M, Bouaziz M, Hammami A.** Emergence of Multidrug-Resistant *Klebsiella Pneumoniae* Isolates Producing VIM-4 Metallo-β-Lactamase, CTX-M-15 Extended-Spectrum β-Lactamase, and CMY-4 AmpC β-Lactamase in a Tunisian University Hospital. Antimicrob Agents Chemother. 2006; 50 (12): 4198-4201.

63. **Chouchani C, Marrakchi R, Henriques I, Correia A.** Occurrence of IMP-8, IMP-10, and IMP-13 Metallo-β-Lactamases Located on Class 1 Integrons and Other Extended-Spectrum β-Lactamases in Bacterial Isolates from Tunisian Rivers. Scand J Infect Dis. 2013; 45 (2): 95-103.

64. **Hammami S, Gautier V, Ghozzi R, Da Costa A, Ben-Redjeb S, Arlet G.** Diversity in VIM-2-encoding class 1 integrons and occasional blaSHV2a carriage in isolates of a persistent, multidrug-resistant *Pseudomonas aeruginosa* clone from Tunis. Clin Microbiol Infect. 2010 ; 16 (2): 189-93.

65. **Hammami S, Boutiba-Ben Boubaker I, Ghozzi R, Saidani M, Amine S, Ben Redjeb S.** Nosocomial outbreak of imipenem-resistant *Pseudomonas aeruginosa* producing VIM-2 metallo-β-lactamase in a kidney transplantation

unit. Diagn Pathol. 2011; 6: 106.

66. **Lahlaoui, H, Poirel L, Barguellil F, M B Moussa, Nordmann P**. Carbapenem-hydrolyzing class D β-lactamase OXA-48 in *Klebsiella pneumoniae* isolates from Tunisia. Eur J Clin Microbiol Infect Dis. 2012; 6: 937-39.

67. **Cuzon G, Naas T, Lesenne A, Benhamou M, Nordmann P**. Plasmid-Mediated Carbapenem-Hydrolysing OXA-48 β-Lactamase in *Klebsiella Pneumoniae* from Tunisia. Int J Antimicrob Agents. 2010 ; 36 (1): 91-93.

68. **Chouchani C, Marrakchi R, Ferchichi L, El Salabi A, Walsh TR.** VIM and IMP Metallo-β-Lactamases and Other Extended-Spectrum β-Lactamases in *Escherichia Coli* and *Klebsiella Pneumoniae* from Environmental Samples in a Tunisian Hospital: VIM AND IMP METALLO-β-LACTAMASES. APMIS. 2011 ; 119 (10): 725-32.

69. **Ben Nasr A, Decré D, Compain F, Genel N, Barguellil N, Arlet G**. Emergence of NDM-1 in Association with OXA-48 in *Klebsiella pneumoniae* from Tunisia. Antimicrob Agents Chemother. 2013; 57 (8): 4089-90.

70. **Saidani M, Hammami S, Kammoun A, Slim A, Boutiba-Ben Boubaker I.** Emergence of Carbapenem-Resistant OXA-48 Carbapenemase- Producing *Enterobacteriaceae* in Tunisia. J Med Microbiol. 2012 ; 61: 1746-49.

71. **Tenney J, Hudson N, Alnifaidy H, Li JTC, Fung KH.** Risk factors for aquiring multidrug-resistant organisms in urinary tract infections: A systematic literature review. Saudi Pharm J. 2016; 26 (5): 678-84.

72. **Shilo S, Assous MV, Lachish T, Kopuit P, Bdolah-Abram T, Yinnon AM et al.** Risk Factors for Bacteriuria with Carbapenem-Resistant *Klebsiella Pneumoniae* and Its Impact on Mortality: A Case-Control Study. Infection. 2013 ; 41(2): 503-9.

73. **Lee DS, Choe HS, Kim HY, Yoo JM, Bae WJ, Cho YH et al.** Role of age and sex in determining antibiotic resistance in febrile urinary tract infections. Int J Infect Dis. 2016; 51: 89-96.

74. **Pavese P.** Nosocomial urinary tract infections: definition, diagnosis, pathophysiology, prevention, treatment. Med Mal Infect. 2003; 33 :266- 74.

75. **Mariappan S, Sekar U, Kamalanathan A**. Carbapenemase-producing *Enterobacteriaceae*: Risk factors for infection and impact of resistance on outcomes. Int J Appl Basic Med Res. 2017; 7 (1): 32-39.

76. **Kaase M, Schimanski S, Schiller R, Beyreiß B, Thürmer A, Steinmann J et al.** Multicentre Investigation of Carbapenemase-Producing *Escherichia Coli* and *Klebsiella Pneumoniae* in German Hospitals. Int J Med Microbiol. 2016; 306 (6): 415-20.

77. **Tang HJ, Hsieh CF, Chang PC, Chen JJ, Lin YH, Lai CC et al.** Clinical

Significance of Community- and Healthcare-Acquired Carbapenem-Resistant *Enterobacteriaceae* Isolates. PLoS One. 2016 ; 11 (3): e0151897.

78. **Dizbay M, Guzel Tunccan O, Karasahin O, Aktas F.** Emergence of carbapenem-resistant *Klebsiella spp.* infections in a Turkish university hospital: epidemiology and risk factors. J Infect Dev Ctries. 2014 ; 8 (1).44-9.

79. **Shah BR, Hux JE.** Quantifying the Risk of Infectious Diseases for People with Diabetes. Diab Care. 2003 ; 26 (2): 510-13.

80. **Nitzan O, Elias M, Chazan B, Saliba W.** Urinary tract infections in patients with type 2 diabetes mellitus: review of prevalence, diagnosis, and management. Diabetes Metab Syndr Obes. 2015; 8:129-36

81. **Lin MY, Lyles-Banks RD, Lolans K, Hines DW, Spear JB, Petrak R et al.** The Importance of Long-Term Acute Care Hospitals in the Regional Epidemiology of *Klebsiella Pneumoniae* Carbapenemase-Producing Enterobacteriaceae. Clin Infect Dis. 2013; 57 (9): 1246-52.

82. **Rossini A, Di Santo SG, Libori MF, Tiracchia V, Balice MP, Salvia A.** Risk Factors for Carbapenemase-Producing *Enterobacteriaceae* Colonization of Asymptomatic Carriers on Admission to an Italian Rehabilitation Hospital. J Hosp Infect. 2016; 92 (1): 78-81.

83. **Kunin CM.** Genitourinary Infections in the Patient at Risk: Extrinsic Risk Factors. Am J Med. 1984; 76 (5A): 131-39.

84. **Nickel JC, Costerton JW, McLean RJ, Olson M.** Bacterial Biofilms: Influence on the Pathogenesis, Diagnosis and Treatment of Urinary Tract Infections. J Antimicrob Chemother. 1994; 33 (suppl A): 31-41.

85. **Jacobsen SM, Stickler DJ, Mobley HL, Shirtliff ME.** Complicated Catheter-Associated Urinary Tract Infections Due to *Escherichia coli* and *Proteus mirabilis*. Clin Microbiol Rev. 2008; 21 (1): 26-59.

86. **Hooton TM, Bradley SF, Cardenas DD, Colgan R, Geerlings SE, Rice JC et al.** Diagnosis, Prevention, and Treatment of Catheter-Associated Urinary Tract Infection in Adults: 2009 International Clinical Practice Guidelines from the Infectious Diseases Society of America. Clin Infect Dis. 2010; 50(5): 625-63.

87. **Smith ZL, Dua A, Saeian K, Ledeboer NA, Graham MB, Aburajab M et al.** A Novel Protocol Obviates Endoscope Sampling for Carbapenem-Resistant *Enterobacteriaceae*: Experience of a Center with a Prior Outbreak. Dig Dis Sci. 2017; 62 (11): 3100-3109.

88. **Faye K.** Veterinary use of antibiotics: impact on bacterial antibiotic resistance in animal and human health. Antibiotiques. 2005 ; 7 (1): 45-52.

89. **Pontiès V, Soing-Altrach S, Savitch Y, Dortet L, NAAS T, Bernet C et al.** Episodes involving enterobacteriaceae producing

carbapenemases in France- National epidemiological review of 31 December 2015. Santé Publique France.

90. **Nordmann P, Cuzon G, Naas T.** The Real Threat of Klebsiella Pneumoniae Carbapenemase-Producing Bacteria. Lancet Infect Dis. 2009 ; 9 (4): 228-36.

91. **de Maio Carrilho CM, de Oliveira LM, Gaudereto J, Perozin JS, Urbano MR, Camargo CH et al.** A prospective study of treatment of carbapenem-resistant *Enterobacteriaceae* infections and risk factors associated with outcome. BMC Infect Dis. 2016; 16 (1): 629.

92. **Alexander EL, Loutit J, Tumbarello M, Wunderink R, Felton T, Daikos G et al.** Carbapenem-Resistant *Enterobacteriaceae* Infections: Results From a Retrospective Series and Implications for the Design of Prospective Clinical Trials. Open Forum Infect Dis. 2017; 4 (2): ofx063.

93. **Lee YC, Hsiao CY, Hung MC, Hung SC, Wang HP, Huang YJ et al.** Bacteremic Urinary Tract Infection Caused by Multidrug-Resistant *Enterobacteriaceae* Are Associated With Severe Sepsis at Admission: Implication for Empirical Therapy. Medicine. 2016; 95 (20): e3694.

94. **Qureshi ZA, Syed A, Clarke LG, Doi Y, Shields RK.** Epidemiology and Clinical Outcomes of Patients with Carbapenem-Resistant *Klebsiella Pneumoniae* Bacteriuria. Antimicrob Agents Chemother. 2014; 58 (6): 3100-04.

95. **El Mahi F.** Epidemiological profile of carbapenemase-producing Enterobacteriaceae diagnosed at CHU Ibn Sina-Rabat. 2013; n:95.

96. **Zilberberg MD, Nathanson BH, Sulham K, Fan W, Shorr AF.** Carbapenem Resistance, Inappropriate Empiric Treatment and Outcomes among Patients Hospitalized with *Enterobacteriaceae* Urinary Tract Infection, Pneumonia and Sepsis. BMC Infect Dis. 2017; 17(1):279.

97. **Xu Y, Gu B, Huang M, Liu H, Xu T, Xia W, Wang T.** Epidemiology of carbapenem resistant *Enterobacteriaceae* (CRE) during 2000-2012 in Asia. J thorac Dis. 2015; 7(3) : 376-85.

98. **Jans B, Catry B, Glupezynsk Y.** Epidemiological surveillance of carbapenem-resistant Enterobacteriaceae (CPE) in Belgium: from January 2012 to June 2014. Scientific Institute of Public Health, Brussels. www.nsih.be; accessed 28 August 2018.

99. **Van Duin D, Cober E, Richter SS, Perez F, Kalayjian RC, Salata RA et al.** Impact of Therapy and Strain Type on Outcomes in Urinary Tract Infections Caused by Carbapenem-Resistant *Klebsiella Pneumoniae*. J Antimicrob Chemother. 2014; 70(4): 1203-11.

100. **Naas T.** The challenges of highly resistant bacteria. http://www.rencontressantepubliquefrance.fr/wp-

content/uploads/2018/06/NAAS.pdf, accessed 27 August 2018.

101. **Mezzatesta ML, La Rosa G, Maugeri G, Zingali T, Caio C, Novelli A et al.** In Vitro Activity of Fosfomycin Trometamol and Other Oral Antibiotics against Multidrug-Resistant Uropathogens. Int J Antimicrob Agents. 2017 ; 49(6): 763-66.

102. **Alexander RT, Marschall J, Tibbetts RJ, Neuner EA, Dunne WM Jr, Ritchie DJ.** Treatment and Clinical Outcomes of Urinary Tract Infections Caused by KPC-Producing Enterobacteriaceae in a Retrospective Cohort. Clin Ther. 2012 ; 34(6): 1314-23.

103. **Papst L, Beovic B, Pulcini C, Durante-Mangoni E, Rodriguez-Baño J, Kaye KS et al.** Antibiotic Treatment of Infections Caused by Carbapenem-Resistant Gram-Negative Bacilli: An International ESCMID Cross-Sectional Survey among Infectious Diseases Specialists Practicing in Large Hospitals. Clin Microbiol Infect.2018; 24(10): 1070-76.

104. **Lee GC, Burgess DS.** Treatment of *Klebsiella Pneumoniae* Carbapenemase (KPC) Infections: A Review of Published Case Series and Case Reports. Ann Clin Microbiol Antimicrob. 2012 ; 11: 32.

105. **Sader HS, Farrell DJ, Jones RN.** Tigecycline Activity Tested against Multidrug-Resistant *Enterobacteriaceae* and *Acinetobacter Spp.* Isolated in US Medical Centers (2005-2009). Diagn Microbiol Infect Dis. 2011; 69(2): 223-27.

106. **Van Duin D, Cober E, Richter SS, Perez F, Kalayjian RC, Salata RA et al.** Residence in Skilled Nursing Facilities is Associated with Tigecycline Non-Susceptibility in Carbapenem-Resistant *Klebsiella pneumoniae.* Infect control hosp epidemiol. 2015; 36(8): 942-48.

107. **Jeong SH, Kim HS, Kim JS, Shin DH, Kim HS, Park MJ et al.** Prevalence and Molecular Characteristics of Carbapenemase-Producing *Enterobacteriaceae* From Five Hospitals in Korea. Ann Lab Med.2016; 36(6): 529-35.

108. **Brust K, Evans A, Plemmons R.** Favourable Outcome in the Treatment of Carbapenem-Resistant *Enterobacteriaceae* Urinary Tract Infection with High-Dose Tigecycline. J Antimicrob Chemother.2014; 69(10): 2875-76.

109. **Gales AC, Jones RN, Sader HS.** Contemporary Activity of Colistin and Polymyxin B against a Worldwide Collection of GramNegative Pathogens: Results from the SENTRY Antimicrobial Surveillance Program (2006-09). J Antimicrob Chemother.2011; 66(9): 2070-74.

110. **Garonzik SM, Li J, Thamlikitkul V, Paterson DL, Shoham S, Jacob J et al.** Population Pharmacokinetics of Colistin Methanesulfonate and Formed Colistin in Critically Ill Patients from a Multicenter Study Provide Dosing Suggestions for Various Categories of Patients. Antimicrob Agents

Chemother.2017; 55(7): 3284-94.

111. **Sandri AM, Landersdorfer CB, Jacob J, Boniatti MM, Dalarosa MG, Falci DR et al**. Population Pharmacokinetics of Intravenous Polymyxin B in Critically Ill Patients: Implications for Selection of Dosage Regimens. Clin Infect Dis.2013; 57(4): 524-31.

112. **Falagas ME, Rafailidis PI, Ioannidou E, Alexiou VG, Matthaiou DK, Karageorgopoulos DE et al.** Colistin Therapy for Microbiologically Documented Multidrug-Resistant Gram-Negative Bacterial Infections: A Retrospective Cohort Study of 258 Patients. Int J Antimicrob Agents.2010; 35(2): 194-99.

113. **Carmeli Y, Akova M, Cornaglia G, Daikos GL, Garau J, Harbarth S et al**. Controlling the spread of carbapenemase-producing Gram-negatives: therapeutic approach and infection control. Clin Microbiol Infect. 2010;16(2):102-11.

114. **Falagas ME, Rafailidis PI, Kofteridis D, Virtzili S, Chelvatzoglou FC, Papaioannou V et al.** Risk factors of carbapenem- resistant *Klebsiella pneumoniae* infections: a matched case control study. J Antimicrob Chemother. 2007; 60(5):1124-30.

115. **Banerjee S, Sengupta M, Sarker TK**. Fosfomycin Susceptibility among Multidrug-Resistant, Extended-Spectrum Beta-Lactamase- Producing, Carbapenem-Resistant Uropathogens. Indian J Urol. 2017 ; 33(2): 149.

116. **Michalopoulos A, Virtzili S, Rafailidis P, Chalevelakis G, Damala M, Falagas ME.** Intravenous Fosfomycin for the Treatment of Nosocomial Infections Caused by Carbapenem-Resistant *Klebsiella Pneumoniae* in Critically Ill Patients: A Prospective Evaluation. Clin Microbiol Infect. 2010 ; 16(2): 184-86.

117. **Daikos GL, Markogiannakis A.** Carbapenemase-Producing *Klebsiella Pneumoniae*: (When) Might We Still Consider Treating with Carbapenems. Clin Microbiol Infect. 2011; 17(8): 1135-41.

118. **Giamarellou H, Galani L, Baziaka F, Karaiskos I.** Effectiveness of a Double-Carbapenem Regimen for Infections in Humans Due to Carbapenemase-Producing Pandrug-Resistant *Klebsiella Pneumoniae*. Antimicrob Agents Chemother. 2013; 57(5): 2388 90.

119. **Tzouvelekis LS, Markogiannakis A, Piperaki E, Souli M, Daikos GL**. Treating Infections Caused by Carbapenemase-Producing *Enterobacteriaceae*. Clin Microbiol Infect. 2014; 20(9): 862-72.

120. **Cattoir, V.** Treatment of infections due to carbapenemase-producing Enterobacteriaceae. J Antiinfec. 2014; 16(3): 99-105.

121. **Mashni O, Nazer L, Le J.** Critical Review of Double-Carbapenem

Therapy for the Treatment of Carbapenemase-Producing *Klebsiella Pneumoniae*. Ann Pharmacother.2018; doi: 10.1177/1060028018790573. [E pub ahead of print].

122. **Murri R, Fiori B, Spanu T, Mastrorosa I, Giovannenze F, Taccari F et al.** Trimethoprim-Sulfamethoxazole Therapy for Patients with Carbapenemase-Producing *Klebsiella Pneumoniae* Infections: Retrospective Single-Center Case Series. Infection. 2017 ; 45(2): 209-13.

123. **Falagas ME, Lourida P, Poulikakos P, Rafailidis PI, Tansarli GS.** Antibiotic Treatment of Infections Due to Carbapenem-Resistant *Enterobacteriaceae*: Systematic Evaluation of the Available Evidence. Antimicrob Agents Chemother. 2014; 58(2): 654-63.

124. **Chang YY, Chuang YC, Siu LK, Wu TL, Lin JC, Lu PL et al.** Clinical Features of Patients with Carbapenem Nonsusceptible *Klebsiella Pneumoniae* and *Escherichia Coli* in Intensive Care Units: A Nationwide Multicenter Study in Taiwan. J Microbiol Immunol Infect. 2015; 48(2): 219-25.

125. **Thaden JT, Pogue JM, Kaye KS.** Role of Newer and ReEmerging Older Agents in the Treatment of Infections Caused by Carbapenem-Resistant *Enterobacteriaceae*. Virulence. 2017 ; 8(4): 40316.

126. Avycaz (Avibactam and Ceftazidime) FDA Approval History. Drugs.com. https://www.drugs.com/history/avycaz.html, accessed on 24 August 2018.

127. **Vazquez JA, González Patzán LD, Stricklin D, Duttaroy DD, Kreidly Z, Lipka J et al.** Efficacy and Safety of Ceftazidime-Avibactam versus Imipenem-Cilastatin in the Treatment of Complicated Urinary Tract Infections, Including Acute Pyelonephritis, in Hospitalized Adults: Results of a Prospective, Investigator-Blinded, Randomized Study. Curr Med Res Opin. 2012 ; 28(12): 1921-31.

128. **Hecker SJ, Reddy KR, Totrov M, Hirst GC, Lomovskaya O, Griffith DC et al.** Discovery of a cyclic boronic acid ß-lactamase inhibitor (RPX7009) with utility vs class a serine carbapenemese. J Med Chem. 2015 ; 58 :3682-92.

129. **Livermore DM, Mushtaq S, Warner M, Woodford N.** In Vitro Activity of Eravacycline against Carbapenem-Resistant *Enterobacteriaceae* and *Acinetobacter Baumannii*. Antimicrob Agents Chemother. 2016; 60(6): 3840-44.

130. **Zhanel GG, Lawson CD, Zelenitsky S, Findlay B, Schweizer F, Adam H et al.** Comparison of the Next-Generation Aminoglycoside Plazomicin to Gentamicin, Tobramycin and Amikacin. Expert Rev Anti Infect Ther. 2012 ; 10(4): 459-73.

131. **Livermore DM, Mushtaq S, Warner M, Zhang JC, Maharjan S,**

Doumith M, Woodford N. Activity of Aminoglycosides, Including ACHN-490, against Carbapenem-Resistant Enterobacteriaceae Isolates. J Antimicrob Chemother. 2011 ; 66(1): 48-53.

132. **Xu L, Sun X, Ma X.** Systematic review and meta-analysis of mortality of patients infected with carbapenem-resistant Klebsiella pneumoniae. Ann Clin Microbiol Antimicrob. 2017 ; 16 :18.

133. **Institut national de santé publique de Québec.** Measures for the prevention and control of carbapenemase-producing Enterobacteriaceae in the environments care.https://www.inspq.qc.ca/sites/default/files/publications/2375_preventi on_control_enterobacteries_carbapenemases.pdf, accessed 29 August 2018.

134. **Naas T.** Epidemiology and prevention of enterobacteria Producers of carbapenemases.http://www.cpias-auvergnerhonealpes.fr/Reseaux/ATB_BMR/Journees/2016/NAAS_BHRe _EPC.pdf, accessed on 28 August 2018.

135. **Tacconelli E, Cataldo MA, Dancer SJ, De Angelis G, Falcone M, Frank U et al.** ESCMID guidelines for the management of the infection control measures to reduce transmission of multidrug-resistant Gram-negative bacteria in hospitalized patients. Clin microbiol infect. 2014; 20:1-55.

136. **Carrër A, Fortineau N, Nordmann P.** Use of the ChromID extended-spectrum beta-lactamase medium for detecting carbapenemase- producing Enterobacteriaceae. J Clin Microbiol. 2010;48:1913-4.

137. **Schechner V, Straus-Robinson K, Schwartz D, Pfeffer I, Tarabeia J, Moskovich R et al.** Evaluation of PCR-based testing for surveillance of KPC-producing carbapenem-resistant members of Enterobacteriaceae family. J Clin Microbiol. 2009;47:3261-5.

Information sheet

Patient's name ;   First name :   File number :

Age ;   Sex: M □ F □   Origin :

Service :   Input: Output :   Length of hospital stay (days)

I. <u>Lifestyle habits :</u>

Socio-economic level: low □ medium   □ high □

Tobacco: no □ yes   □

Alcohol: no □ yes   □

Risk behaviours/addiction: no □ ord (please specify ;   )

                    Notion of recent trip): no □ yes □ (please specify -country :

                              -duration of stay :

                              -ttt during the stay: no □ yes □

                              -hospitalisation: no □ yes □

II. <u>Medical history :</u>

1) History of chronic illness

-Diabetes :	no □	yes □
-HTA :	non□	yes □
-Dyslipidemia :	non□	yes □
-COPD :	noû	yes □
-Other respiratory pathology :	non□	yes □ (please specify :)
-Heart failure :	noi!	yes □
-Renal insufficiency: no □		yes □
-Autoimmune disease:	no^l	yes □ (please specify:)
-Progressive neoplasia :	noi]	yes □ (please specify:)
-Malignant haemopathies : noi]		yes □ (please specify:)
-radiotherapy/chemotherapy:	no[]	yes □
-ttt immunosuppressant : no□		yes □
-Long-term corticosteroid therapy: no□		yes □
-Neurological bladder:	no Q]	or□
-Others :		yes □

2) <u>Urological history :</u>

yes Y (specify location   )

- renal colic: no ∏   yes □

-Known urinary lithiasis: no Q   yes □

-prostate adenoma: no □   yes □ (type of :   )

-Urethritis and/or prostatitis: no []   oui □

-malformative uropathy: no □   no □ oui □ (specify duration:)

-urinary catheterisation: no []   no □ oui □ (specify cause:)

If yes, specify the type of survey: -transitory :   no□ yes □ (specify cause:)

-permanent : - intermittent :

<u>**3) History of infections :**</u>

***Urinary tract infections :**   no □ yes □

if yes, specify :

Date	Type of urinary infection (cystitis, PNA, male UTI)	Germ involved	ATB prescribed (molecule, dose, duration)	Inpatient or outpatient treatment	Length of hospital stay	Possible complications

***Infections other than urinary tract infection:** no D yes □

Type of infection	date	ATB (molecule, dose, duration)	hospitalisation		
			no	yes	
				service	Length of stay

<u>**History of hospitalisation in the last 6 months:**</u> no □ yes □

<u>**4)**</u>

If yes, specify : - department :

-duration of hospitalisation :

<u>**5) History of surgery in the last 6 months:**</u> noti yes □

If yes, specify type :

<u>**6) Previous use of antibiotics (in the last 6 months):**</u> no □ yes □

If yes, please specify: -molecules and duration of treatment: -peniA O   (duration :)

- C3G   O   (duration   :   )
- Fluoroquinolones I-I   (duration :   )
- Carbapenems □ (duration :   )
- Others : O

a--

-compliance: good □poor   □

<u>**7) Foreign material fitted in the last 6 months:**</u> no Q yes Q

(If yes, specify type: urinary   catheter□

Central venous catheter □

Arteriovenous fistula □

Osteosynthesis material □

Others :

III. <u>Reason for hospitalisation :</u>

***Inpatient department : *Bias: URG Q C.ext Q Transfer LP doctor**

IV. <u>Entrance examination :</u>

General condition :   T°= TA= Fc= FR= Dextro=

Urine dipstick :(Au : Gu : L : N :   )

Presence of a heart murmur: no □yes   □

Presence of respiratory impairment: no □yes   □ (specify:)

SGC= /15; state of consciousness: normal □altered   ]

Lumbar shaking pain: no Q yes Q

TR: normal D prostate enlarged□   sensitive prostate O

pSOFA score :

Another anomaly:

V. <u>Additional tests:</u>

1) <u>Biology</u>

*NFS: (HB=   g/dl;   VGM= ; TCMH= ; CCMH=

GB=   /mm^3 ; with PNN= /mm^3 and lymphocytes= / mm^3

Plq=   /mm^3 °

* TP=   TCK=   fibrinogen=

*Urea=   mmol/l Créat= umol/l

*ALAT=   UI/l   ASAT= UI/l

*CRP=   mg/l

*GDS: (PH=   ;   PaO2= ; PaCO2= ; HCO3-=

SaO2= ; Lactates=)

*Blood cultures (number=) :

Blood culture number	Culture		
	negative	Positive	
		Germ	antibiogram
n°1			
n°2			
n°3			

*ECBU:(L= /mm^3 ; H= /mm^3 ; culture= Antibiogram :

*Other direct debits :

-pus sampling   □ (culture :   antibiogram :   )

-culture of the tip of the bladder catheter □ (culture :   antibiogram :   )

-Growing a piece of KT   □ (culture :   antibiogram :   )

-ECBC   □ (culture :   antibiogram :   )

-other :

2) <u>Radiology :</u>

-Radiothorax: normal O   pathological O (specify abnormalities ;   )

-AUSP :   no done EJ   done Π (if done specify ; normad lithiasû)

-Renal and bladder/vesicoprostatic ultrasound: not done □ done □

*kidney and bladder: -normal □

-pathological O (nephromegaly □ dilatation of CPtfJ lithiasisJ

Decreased cortico-medullary differentiation □

Cortical hypoechogenicity □ Renal abscess □

Sequelae of PNAJ Bladder thickening □

Other □

*prostatic: -normal □

-pathological □(increased prostate size □ calcifications^

Other □)

-CT: not doneQ done 0 (if done, specify; normal ∏ pathological []   )

-other :

VI. <u>Treatment</u>

<u>1) Antibiotic therapy</u>: monotherapy Q combination of TBAs Q

Molecule			
Dose			
Track			
Duration			

*switch: no□ yes □

If yes, specify : - the deadline :

-the cause: -failure (unfavourable evolution, complication...) Q

adaptation to antibiotic susceptibility testing: ∏ - de-escalation].

- climbing □

-        adverse effectsD (please specify:)

-        drug interactions □

-terms and conditions

Molecule			
Dose			
Route of administration			
Duration			

<u>2) Other treatments</u>

VII. <u>Developments</u>

Favourable Unfavourable

1/ if favourable, specify :

-apyrexia time (days) :

- change in functional signs: - regression (time ;   )∏

-disappearance (time ;   )□

-Output: noO yes □

Molecule			
Shape			
Dose			
Duration			

Backtracking: no D yes □ (follow-up time:)

2/ if unfavourable :

-÷ complication: □

(The complication is related to: -infection □ (specify:)

- Prolonged dorsal decubitus □

-decompensation of an underlying defect ∏

-÷ death: □ -delay: - cause:

VIII. <u>Cost</u>

- **Cost of hospitalisation =**
- **Cost of antibiotic therapy =**

Summary

The emergence of carbapenem-resistant enterobacterial urinary tract infections is an alarming health problem, particularly in resource-limited countries. The aim of our work is to describe the epidemioclinical, paraclinical, therapeutic and evolutionary features of these infections, as well as the factors involved in the selection of these resistant strains. This is a retrospective descriptive study including all patients hospitalised in the departments of the Taher Sfar Mahdia University Hospital (from January 2015 to April 2018) who had presented with a carbapenem-resistant Enterobacteriaceae urinary tract infection. Twenty-three patients were enrolled. They had an average age of 57.3 years with a sex ratio M/F= 0.77. The majority of patients (47.8%) were admitted to a medical intensive care unit. The infection was healthcare-associated in 56.5% of cases. The main risk factors for acquiring ERC were: previous antibiotic therapy (beta-lactams), previous hospitalisation, an invasive procedure in the previous six months, and a history of urinary tract infection in the previous year. A univariate analysis of the different risk factors according to the bacterial species isolated showed an association between bladder catheterisation and carbapenem-resistant *Klebsiella pneumoniae* UTI ($p = 0.026$). The clinical picture was severe in the majority of cases (69.6%): a deterioration in general condition and consciousness in 69.6% and 56.5% of cases respectively. Eight patients (34.7%) were in sepsis or septic shock. Biologically, hyperleukocytosis and elevated CRP were found in 82.6% and 95.6% of cases respectively. The germs isolated were *Klebsiella pneumoniae* (69.5%), *Enterobacter cloacae* (26.0%) and *Enterobacter aerogenes* (4.3%). The antibiotic susceptibility rate of the isolated strains was: 100% for colistin, 87% for amikacin and fosfomycin, 56.5% for tigecycline, 17.4% for sulfa/trimethoprim and 13% for gentamicin. A combination of antibiotics was indicated in 19 cases (82.6%). The most commonly prescribed antibiotic combinations were colimycin + tigecycline and tigecycline + amikacin. Univariate analysis showed that the prescription of tigecycline was significantly associated with an unfavourable outcome *($p = 0.032$)*. Outcome also depended on the severity of the clinical picture: severe sepsis or septic shock was significantly associated with death *($p = 0.026$)*. The average cost of treating these infections was 3334.4 DT +/- 2844.9. Carbapenem-resistant urinary tract infections are a health problem in Tunisia. Intervention strategies must be integrated and target decision-makers, prescribers and patients alike.

Title :   Carbapenem resistantent erobacteriaceae in urinary tract infections

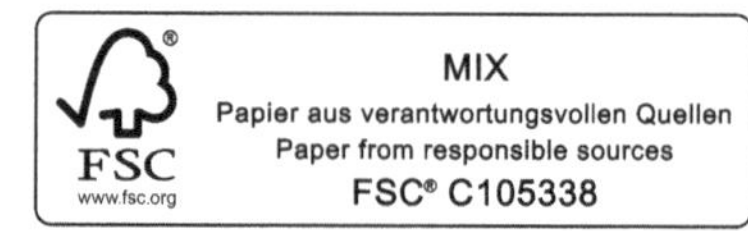

Printed by Books on Demand GmbH, Norderstedt / Germany